CANDIDA HEALTH

THROUGH

LIVING FOODS

LALITA SALAS

Requests for permission should be addressed to:

Ann Wigmore Institute Publishing
P.O. Box 429
Rincón, Puerto Rico 00677
Fax: 787.868.2430

Author: Claudia (Lalita) Salas
Cover Design: Pablo Montes O'Neill
Book Design and Project Director: Michele Jarvey
Photographs: Luis Marin
Printed in the United States
ISBN: 978-0-615-23802-9
Library of Congress Control Number: 2008933809

This book is not intended as a scientific guide for overcoming Candida overgrowth. This book is a result of many years of reading the research work of others, personal experiences and personal experimentation of the author. Because there is always some risk involved, the author and publisher are not responsible for any adverse effects or consequences resulting from the use of any of the suggestions, preparations or procedures in this book. Please do not use this book if you are unwilling to assume the risk. Feel free to consult a physician or other qualified health professionals. Living Foods Lifestyle® is a registered trademark co-owned by the Ann Wigmore Foundation and the Ann Wigmore Natural Health Institute.

This book is dedicated to:

The memory of Dr. Ann Wigmore my teacher, my mentor, my guide into the path of self-healing

To all the students that come to the institute looking for their long time lost connection with the inner self

To those who have inspired me with their quest for knowledge about Candida Health; all hold a special place in my heart **–Lalita Salas**

Contents

Foreword   1

Introduction   3

What is Candida   5

What Causes Candida   11

What are the Symptoms   15

Reaching an Ecological Balance   17

Lalita's Personal Struggle   27

Food Sources   39

Living Foods   41

Breakfast   45

    Amaranth Creamy Cereal   45
    Berry Flake Cereal   46
    Breakfast Smoothie   47
    Living Quinoa Cereal   48
    Buckwheat Apple Cereal   49

Appetizers & Side Dishes   51

    Almond Sauce   51
    Basic Pumpkin Seed Paté   51
    Blended Salsa   52
    Guacamole   53
    Zucchini Hummus   54

Soups	55
Cucumber Soup	55
Energy Soup	56
Celery Soup	58
Avocado Chowder	59
Vegetable Soup	60
Salads	**61**
Avocado Sprout Salad	61
Simple Healthy Salad	61
Creamy Cucumber Salad	62
Tabouli Salad	63
Tossed Green Salad	64
Entrées	**65**
Zucchini Spaghetti	65
Almond Pâté	66
Pizza	68
Garden Burgers	70
Stuffed Avocados	72
Desserts	**73**
Almond Strawberry Cream	73
Apple Pie	74
Sunflower Cherry Cream	76
Quinoa Raspberry Delight	76
Avocado Strawberry Pudding	77
Crackers, Chips and Bread	**79**
Zucchini Flax Crackers	79
Buckwheat Flax Crackers	80
Vegetable Flax Crackers	81
Quinoa Chips	82
Quinoa Flax Bread	84
Sauces and Dressings	**87**
Marinara Sauce	87
Parmesan Cheese	88
Carrot Sauce	88
Tomatillo Sauce	89
Apple Ginger Dressing	90
Basic Dressing	90
Carrot Ginger Dressing	91

Milk   93

    Seed Milk   93
    Almond Milk   93

Cultured Foods   95

    Quinoa Rejuvelac   96
    Cabbage Rejuvelac   97
    Veggie Kraut   98
    Seed Cheese   100
    Yogurt   102

Equipment List   103

Sprouting Chart   107

Testimonials   111

Closing Thoughts   114

Acknowledgments   115

Author's Note   119

About Ann Wigmore   123

References   127

Foreword

It is an honor for me to introduce a book that completely embraces the Ann Wigmore Living Foods Lifestyle® concept.

Lalita Salas has been my friend and confidant since 1991; together we are program-directors of the Ann Wigmore Natural Health Institute (AWNHI) in Puerto Rico. Lalita is an instructor and Living Foods Lifestyle coach and practitioner. She is also a yoga instructor, colon hydro therapist, elementary school teacher and a licensed pharmacist.

The Living Foods Lifestyle® foods consist primarily of organically grown vegetables and sprouts, fruits, nuts, seeds, energy soup, cultured and blended foods and wheatgrass juice. In this book, Lalita spotlights living food recipes geared to prevent or reduce the cause of Candida without losing focus of the necessity for tasty yet easy to digest nourishment.

Many of our students and guests at the AWNHI have expressed an interest in obtaining more information on Candida. People want more knowledge to enable them to combat this "illusive" disease through informed food and lifestyle choices.

Approximately 15 years ago I attended a Candida support group in San Francisco CA. I discovered that there seemed to be no solid information on how to avoid this disease naturally with a healthy food program. Everyone was simply exchanging information on medication that might work. My own knowledge was

Foreword

limited and I felt as though I could not help these people. I remember thinking that the air in the room felt thick with toxins.

I have observed Lalita's continuous research and self experimentation searching for a natural solution to overcome her personal challenge with Candida. Lalita Salas is a faithful follower of the living foods lifestyle leading us through her example.

I have been an "official taster" of many recipes being offered in this book therefore feel authorized to endorse these selections as tasty delicacies. These recipes were written by Lalita and prepared by our own specialty chef Manuel Acevedo.

In this book Lalita Salas takes us to a new dimension in the fight against Candida using living foods for living bodies. Lalita believes as Hippocrates taught. "Let food be your medicine". As you learn how to prepare these enjoyable living meals designed specifically for Candida challenges you are on the path to taking responsibility for your health.

Welcome to Candida Health Through Living Foods. I invite you to turn the page and begin this wonderful and exciting journey towards better health!

With Love and Friendship,

Leola A. Brooks

Introduction

I felt an urgency to share with everyone the knowledge I had gained about how and why our bodies could become so depleted. When our bodies become depleted it seems almost impossible to reverse the composting process going on within us. When those feelings were happening to me I would remember a saying from Ann Wigmore, "Nothing is impossible when we give nature a chance."

When people are so depleted and filled with pain they tend to get confused about the needs of their own body. They often find it hard to believe that changing their food choices will help cure them. It is natural to feel discouragement and resistance to giving up our "comfort" food that seems to be such a major part of our identity.

I tried to include nutritional alternatives to some common comfort foods in these recipe choices. These living foods taste great, are ecstatically pleasing and can help with the fight against an overgrowth of Candida in your body.

"Human beings, the potentially highest form of life expression on this planet have built the vast pharmaceutical industry for the central purpose of poisoning the lowest form of life on the planet--germs! One of the biggest tragedies of human civilization is the precedence of chemicals over nutrition." -**Dr. Richard Murray**

What is Candida

In the most basic terms, Candida, when out of control, is an overgrowth of fungus in our bodies caused by a complete ecological imbalance within us. Because of this imbalance in our bodies, our fungus or Candida is busy doing its job trying very hard to compost or recycle us. The fungus or fungi are one of earth's natural recyclers; they are an important part of nature's composting cycle. A Candida overgrowth is nature's messenger screaming to us for help, almost begging us to do something for our body's well being.

Fungi are one of the earth's most powerful recyclers, they are a very important requirement in life. Mold and Yeast belong in the fungus family and often the terms fungus, mold, and yeast are used interchangeably and although both mold and yeast belong in the fungus family, there are distinctions between them.

- Yeast reproduce by asexual budding and anaerobic respiration or fermentation (they can live without oxygen). Candida belongs to the yeast variety of fungi as opposed to the mold variety.
- Mold reproduces both sexually and asexually with hyphae and are primarily aerobic respirators (they cannot live without oxygen.)

Fungus varieties can be very different, while some feed off dead organisms making them nature's own garbage disposal, other types such as parasitic fungus feed off live organisms. These pathogenic or parasitic fungi cause plant, animal and human diseases such as; athlete's foot, swimmer's ear, ringworm, dandruff, valley fever, fingernail and toenail infections, rosacea, yeast and urinary tract infections. The fungi sprout from spore and grow as filaments termed hyphae. Hyphae from individual fungus cells interconnect with hyphae from other cells, forming one large organism termed the mycelium. Hyphae extend at their tips. The tips growth enables fungi to grow continuously into fresh zones of nutrients. This growth pattern is precisely how fungi spread inside the body throughout an imbalanced terrain.

Fungi live in damp environments allowing the hyphae to absorb nutrients that are dissolved in water. The hyphae absorb simple, soluble nutrients (glucose, amino acids, etc) through their walls and release extracellular enzymes, which in turn degrade or digest more complex nutrients. We eat our food, then digest and absorb it; fungi digest their food outside of their own body, then absorb it.

I again refer to the idea that fungi are inside of us to compost us because our body is not in balance with nature. The fungi are simply doing their recycling job because that is what they were designed to do. In Natures grand plan each cell in the plant and animal kingdom has a specific job to do to maintain an ecological balance on this planet.

We become a fungus host and the fungus injects its host with toxins (disease) for survival purposes (to dissolve and digest it or us). The toxins and enzymes that the fungi produce can disable, kill and then dissolve their food sources or host so that the nutrients can be assimilated. When we become the food source for fungus, we are slowly being dissolved and killed. Most cases of fungus and yeast infection are caused by Candida, primarily Candida Albicans, and Candida Aspergillus.

What is Candida

Dr. Ann used to say: Most people think that disease comes from some mysterious place outside the body. When asked what causes disease, most people will answer that germs, bacteria and other "bad guys" are the culprits. Many people do not understand that the "bad guys" (bacteria, germs and parasites) are everywhere in nature. They are a natural part of the ecological balancing process, always on stand-by in nature and within us. They become active only when there is decay, actually it is decay and death that they thrive on. When something is not healthy and does not meet up to Mother Nature's standards, it is "composted" by clean–up crews like germs, bacteria and parasites. That is how a Candida overgrowth operates in our bodies; like a cleanup crew trying to compost the unhealthy or decaying materials. Candida is not the "bad guy" Candida is just doing its job and trying to get rid of the decay.

As an experiment, Dr. Ann once put some food inside an airtight container. About a month later, she opened the container and discovered organisms such as worms and microbes digesting the decaying material. Where did they come from? They were inherently present from the beginning but were inactive or dormant because there was no decay when the jar was sealed. Dr. Ann's observation was supported by research from many medical doctors.

What is Candida

Antoine Bechamp (1816-1908) discovered tiny organisms he called microzyma which are present in all things; animals, vegetables and minerals, whether living or dead. Although these microzymas are present in the tissue and blood of all living organism, they remain quiescent and harmless. However, in a diseased body, they become pathological bacteria and viruses. These microzyma, including specific bacteria, could take on a number of forms during the host's life cycle depending (as Claude Bernard contended) primarily on the chemistry of their environment, the biological terrain or simply stated, the condition of the host. In other words he believed there was no single cause of disease, instead disease results when these organisms change form (the pleomorphic or multi form germ theory) or become toxic according to the terrain of the host. Bechamp had built upon and extended Bernard's idea, developing his own theory of health and disease.

Bad bacteria, viruses and fungi are merely the forms assumed by the microzymas when there is a condition or terrain that favors disease and these "bad" microzyma themselves give off toxic byproducts, further contributing to a weakened terrain. A weakened terrain naturally becomes vulnerable to external harmful bacteria. So, our bodies in effect are mini-ecosystems or biological terrains in which nutritional status, level of toxicity and PH or acid/alkaline balance play key roles.

Dr Gunther Enderlein (1872-1968) confirmed the existence of these microzymas (he referred to them as Protit–microorganisms) and concluded that they change their form according to the conditions of the blood. The Protits are very small (.001 micron) and form a colloidal

8

What is Candida

energetic field, not only within our cells, but also in extra-cellular fluid, the lymph nodes and the blood. This Protit colloidal field is affected by their environment. When people become too acidic, the natural fermentation process in the body is accelerated and the living colloidal energetic field turns into an unhealthy field.

Dr Louis Pasteur the creator of the "germ theory" in relation to disease stated, "Disease arises from micro-organisms outside the body, microorganisms are generally to be guarded against, every disease is associated with a particular microorganism. Microorganisms are primarily causal agents, therefore disease can strike anybody." Although reportedly on his deathbed Pasteur declared, "Claude Bernard was right, the microbe is nothing, the terrain is everything."

At about the time Pasteur was promoting his monomorphic (or single form) germ theory, a contemporary by the name of **Dr. Claude Bernard** (1813-1878) was developing the theory that the body's ability to heal was dependent on its general condition or internal environment. Thus disease occurred only when the terrain or internal environment of the body became favorable to germs. Pasteur and Bernard were in constant controversy over the cause of disease, but in the end, it was evident that Pasteur concurred with Claude Bernard.

In Conclusion :
These microzymas are present in the tissues and blood of all living organisms where they remain quiescent and harmless. Only in a diseased or unbalanced body, will these microzymas become pathological bacteria, viruses or fungi. In a healthy body microzymas form healthy cells. Even with all this knowledge, humans still struggle with bacteria, viruses and fungi instead of simply cleaning up the toxic terrain inside our bodies.

Over 30-years ago a doctor prescribed a very strong antibiotic for an ear infection my 3-month old son had developed. When I questioned, "Why would you give such a strong antibiotic to a baby?" He responded, "Years ago doctors would never give this strong of a medication even to an adult. The problem is that bacteria have become resistant to the antibiotics and we have to find stronger and stronger medicine."

At the time it seemed to me that we were fighting an endless war.

What Causes Candida

It seems that we are like children but without the natural wisdom of children. We play with natural resources without control or respect and in turn, nature acts like a mother to us, never complaining until she is completely exhausted. We learn as much as we can from nature then we use our vast intelligence to take that information and work in our laboratories trying to reproduce things like vitamins, minerals and "natural" healthy food choices. **When in many cases we have moved so far away from Mother Nature with processed, refined and manufactured foods that she responds to us in different and strange ways;** it is as though we have violated her with our chemicals and other poisonous toxins.

Elements Influencing Yeast Overgrowth
A yeast overgrowth can be the result of a combination of many things. Candida is a member of the normal flora of the skin, mouth, vagina and stool. They are normally well tolerated by those with a healthy immune system, however when the Candida yeast increase in number, they create additional stress to the immune system, which in turn can lead to an overgrowth. The growth of yeasts are normally controlled by the presence of Acidophilus and other beneficial bacteria. When these beneficial or friendly bacteria become depleted, an overgrowth is usually inevitable.

Refined and processed sugar in the diet can be one of the greatest contributors to Candida overgrowth. Unnatural sugar is one of yeast's favorite foods!

What Causes Candida

Common elements include:

- Antibiotics which are frequently given for urinary and ear infections, sinusitis, bronchitis and other infections (Candida overgrowth can be triggered at a very young age when children are first being treated with antibiotics.)
- Chronic viral infections
- Dehydration
- Excessively fast bowel transit time (chronic diarrhea)
- Heavy metal toxicity
- Hypothyroidism
- Immune-damaging illnesses such as diabetes
- Medication such as cortisone, or corticosteroids, often prescribed for skin conditions like rashes, eczema or psoriasis, and for rheumatoid arthritis
- Oral contraceptives
- Polluted environment (air, water, soil)
- Processed refined sugars
- Radiation
- Typical American Diet: high fat, high sugar, high starch, nutrient-poor diet, acid forming foods
- Ulcer medications targeted to reduce the amount of acid in the stomach and intestines

Candida is seen in people who are dying of cancer or other very serious diseases. Babies may be born with an internal fungal infection that has been passed to them from their mother. Babies can also develop a Candida diaper rash that tends to be in the deepest part of the creases in the groin and buttocks areas. The rash is usually very red with a clearly-defined border and small red spots close to the large patches. Another common form of Candida in children is thrush on the gums that look like little white spots or cottage cheese.

In his book "Optimal Wellness" Dr. Ralph Golan writes, "Wherever the yeast colonize, they cause symptoms, whether an itchy anus or vagina, diarrhea, heartburn or sore throat. They can also colonize in the sinuses and trigger sinus, ear and eye symptoms. If the damage is to the skin, then itching, hives, and rashes are likely reactions. The yeast release toxic by-products that enter and circulate throughout the bloodstream and cause disturbances in organs and tissues distant from the growing yeast colonies. Such diverse conditions as bronchial asthma, mucous colitis, schizophrenia, lupus, sinusitis, premenstrual tension, bleeding between periods, and recurrent infections can all be caused by tissue injury from yeast."

A yeast impaired immune system can become so confused that it can produce antibodies that attack the body's own tissues and other substances not normally considered foreign matter in the body such as food. The immune system consists partially of Lymphocytes. These Lymphocytes have other types of cells but we will focus on the **B**-cells and **T**-cells. The purpose of the **B**-cells is to create antibodies to attack foreign organisms or substances. The **T**-cells which are the **S**-Suppressor cells and the **H**–Helper cells are the communicators to the **B**-cells. This is how it works; the **H**elper-cells send a message to the **B**-cells telling them to release antibodies to fight diseased or bad cells. When the job is finished, the **S**uppressor-cells send the message to the **B**-cells to stop producing antibodies. The **B**-cells left unchecked can go wild and make antibodies to attack substances that ordinarily would not be considered foreign matter or in need of recycling. These **B**-cells remain unchecked when the immune system is damaged from the toxins produced by an overgrowth of yeast. When this happens, the Suppressor cells are inhibited from sending the message to the **B**-cells to stop producing antibodies, so in turn, these unchecked **B**-cells keep producing antibodies that busily begin destroying healthy cells.

People with Candida have a lower than normal tolerance for ordinarily safe levels of common chemicals such as; gas fumes, oil fumes, cleaning fluids, chlorine, perfume and pesticide residue on produce. The yeast syndrome has been related to autoimmune diseases such as rheumatoid arthritis, multiple sclerosis and scleroderma. Candidacies (which is an infection caused by Candida fungi) is now attributed to be a significant cause of Chronic Fatigue Syndrome, sudden childhood Autism and Attention Deficit Disorder (ADD).

Candida can cause inflammation in the small bowel which in turn can cause incomplete digestion and poor assimilation of nutrients.

This inflammation creates a condition called Leaky Gut Syndrome where large undigested food molecules and other foreign substances enter the circulatory system triggering food allergies and other intolerances.

Candidacies is a big recycling process, which we can control, we simply need to re-store the lost micro-ecological balance in our bodies. As you continue reading, you will find out that this can be done by controlling not only our diets, but our lifestyle as a whole.

What are the Symptoms

There are many symptoms or conditions that indicate an overgrowth of Candida in our bodies. There are so many in fact that people become confused trying to understand the relationship that each of these symptoms has with Candida. But please be honest with yourself. If you have one or more of these symptoms, even if the symptoms come and go but always reoccur under certain circumstances, it is time to pay attention to the warning signs your body is giving you.

"Candida is an elusive thing, and society as a whole is just beginning to open up to this Candida subject."
–Leola Brooks

What are the Symptoms

Candida Albicans Symptoms:
- Allergies
- Brain Fog – difficulty concentrating
- Chronic Fatigue - especially after eating
- Chronic Bad Breath
- Cold Hands or feet or general chilliness
- Depression
- Dry Mouth
- Feeling light headed after minimal alcohol or certain foods
- Fungus growth in the nail area
- Gastrointestinal problems
  Bloating
  Chronic Diarrhea
  Constipation
  Gas
  Heartburn
  Impotence
  Intestinal cramps
- Hypothyroid symptoms
- Insomnia
- Irritability when hungry
- Joint pain or swelling
- Leaky Gut Syndrome
- Memory loss
- Severe mood swings
- Mentally disturbed or spaced out
- Muscle aches
- Premenstrual Syndrome
- Prostatitis
- Psoriasis
- Rectal Itching
- Severe Premenstrual Syndrome
- Shaking
- Recurrent vaginal or urinary infections

Reaching an Ecological Balance

Food is the key to reaching the perfect ecological balance. I have found that positive results occur much faster with the exclusive use of Living Foods during the rebalancing process.

Vegetables are one of the most treasured gifts that nature has to offer us to assist with this delicate balancing act. Vegetables are rich with vitamins and minerals which are extremely important to the healing process of the body. Non-starchy vegetables are recommended to help with the restoration of the body's micro-ecological balance and to help your body stop the overgrowth of Candida.

Non-Starchy Vegetables:

- Arugula
- Asparagus
- Beet Greens
- Bok Choy
- Broccoli
- Brussels Sprouts
- Cabbage
- Cauliflower
- Celery
- Chives
- Collard Greens
- Cucumbers
- Dandelion Greens
- Endive
- Escarole
- Fennel
- Green Beans
- Jicama
- Kale
- Lamb's Quarters
- Lettuces
- Mustard Greens
- Okra
- Parsley
- Radishes
- Red Bell Peppers
- Scallions
- Spinach
- Sprouts
- Swiss Chard
- Turnips
- Watercress
- Yellow Squash
- Zucchini

Reaching an Ecological Balance

I recommend blending the tender green vegetables into energy soup, but you can also enjoy them in a fresh salad. Try to eat a bowl of Energy Soup at least twice a day during the restoration process. Blended foods offer such a high concentration of nutrients in an easy-to-digest form obviously making nutrients from blended foods much easier for the body to absorb.

Some of the hard to digest vegetables like broccoli, cauliflower, carrots and cabbage are great when prepared as Veggie-kraut; this process makes them easier on the digestive system and also provides a good source of lactobacilli, a friendly bacterium which aids in the digestion process. Another way to prepare some of the harder to digest vegetables would be simply to process in a blender or dehydrate at 115F for a few hours. Harder greens like collard greens, kale, etc. are easier to digest when blended or softened by massaging with a bit of mashed avocado, mixed with celery powder and lemon, then marinated for 1 hour. (I love these greens prepared this way and then diced very fine and mixed in with a salad.)

I refer to dehydrated and ground celery as celery powder which should not be confused with "Celery Salt" that can be purchased in a grocery store.

Sauerkraut or Veggie-kraut not only supplies the body with lactobacilli, but is also an excellent food to help control food cravings.

Squash; both yellow summer squash and zucchini are great for Living Food Lasagna and Spaghetti.

Reaching an Ecological Balance

Vegetables to be eaten in Moderation:
- Carrots - Root vegetables have a moderate to high glycemic level however, when cooked the composition changes and the glycemic level increases substantially.
- Tomatoes and be used occasionally but never eat them cooked because the natural acids become inorganic and can be very detrimental to the body creating stress on the kidney and bladder.
- Avocados can be used sparingly because the oil content is a little high for Candida sufferers.

Vegetables to Avoid:
- Beets are very high in sugar.
- Eggplant, although they do have some good qualities, they also have a high acidic level which can be an irritant to the nervous system for the sensitive terrain of a Candida sufferer.
- Green Bell Peppers because they are not completely ripe therefore have not developed all the nutrients making them an incomplete food.
- Mung Bean sprouts can be moldy and should be avoided.
- Mushrooms are too acid forming and full of micro-toxins.
- Russet Potatoes, Sweet Potatoes and Yams are all too high in starch.

Reaching an Ecological Balance

Herbs:

The best way to eat herbs is fresh. They have the best flavor when they are fresh and you do not have to worry about fungus or mold like you do with dried spices as they get old. Basil, chives, dill, ginger, oregano etc can add a delicious flavor to food but I recommend using these in small quantities so as not to overpower the wonderful natural flavors of your fresh vegetable dishes.

Stevia is a sweet herb; it is approximately 300 times sweeter than sugar. Stevia is originally from North and South America and grows wild in Brazil and Paraguay. According to research, stevia does not raise blood sugar levels so is a good sweetener for people with diabetes and hypoglycemia. It is antifungal and considered very good to help balance the pancreas. You can buy stevia in most health food stores in a white powder or liquid form. I recommend purchasing the unrefined green powder stevia. For the best tasting and most health conscious choice you may grow your own fresh leafy stevia.

Reaching an Ecological Balance

Fruits:

Fruits are a very controversial subject for most people because after all, nature provided us with fruits that are filled with nutrients. Many people wonder; how can we change our diet so much AND cut out the fruits? I do not recommend cutting out all fruit, but I do recommend people completely eliminating the moderate and high glycemic fruits during the restoration process. We also need to take into consideration just how micro-toxic the person is when removing fruits or adding them back into the diet. The fruits in level one are healing and can be used by everyone and most people can tolerate the fruits in level two without a problem. I recommend completely removing fruits in levels three and four during the initial Candida cleansing phase. The level of micro-toxicity in your body will help determine how long before you can begin to incorporate fruits from the next level back into your diet. One young lady with Candida had a side effect of Psoriasis that she had been suffering with for years. She followed the program strictly and decided to add one green apple a day. Within two months she healed her Psoriasis completely even with the addition of one serving of a level three fruit. The key element is to listen to your body and do what is best for your personal healing journey because each person will be slightly different in this process. Fruits should always be eaten fresh and unsweetened. Canned or processed fruits should never be used.

When people are in a composting process due to a chronic degenerative disease they will have a significant amount of Candida. A Living Food diet including lemons and limes usually helps the person improve within a two or three month period. After that initial balancing process one may gradually move into the low glycemic fruit group and then again gradually move into the moderate group only using the highest glycemic fruit group occasionally.

Dr Gabriel Cousens's book, "Rainbow Green Live-food Cuisine" pg: 32 provides a list of researched glycemic fruits and vegetables. During my cleansing experience with Candida, I followed Dr. Cousens's recommendations regarding glycemic fruits.

Level One
- Lemons
- Limes

Level Two - Low Glycemic Fruits
- Blueberries
- Cherries
- Cranberries
- Coconut Water
- Soft Coconut Pulp
- Grapefruit
- Gojiberries
- Raspberries
- Strawberries

Level Three – Moderate Glycemic Fruits
- Apples
- Blackberries
- Oranges
- Peaches
- Pears
- Plums
- Pomegranates

Level Four – High Glycemic Fruits
- Apricots
- Bananas
- Dates
- Figs
- Grapes
- Kiwi
- Mangos
- Melons
- Papaya
- Pineapple
- Raisins

It seems that people with chronic diseases need to be between levels one, two, and three for a period of up to six months to reverse the process according to Dr. Cousens's experiences with patients. A person with cancer could take up to two years or more to permanently turn off the composting button.

In my personal experience it took a year. I believe it was because I moved into the low glycemic group followed with the moderate level slowly, but I jumped into the high glycemic group quickly and felt the symptoms return almost immediately. Like I stated before, my body responds the best with low glycemic fruits and a minimum amount of the moderate group while only occasionally eating high glycemic fruits.

GRAINS:
Gluten-free grains are the best choice because they do not promote Candida. People with a chronic degenerative disease should remove grains entirely from their diet for a period of two to three months or consume very small amounts but only occasionally.

- Amaranth
- Buckwheat
- Millet
- Quinoa

I can not stress enough the importance of soaking and sprouting grains. This makes them easier to digest and much less acid and mucus forming. I do not recommend eating an abundance of grains, it is more important to focus your food consumption on greens and include only 15% or less of grains into your diet.

According to Dr. Cousens, in his book Rainbow Green Live-Food Cuisine pg 23; "Most grains create acidity and are associated with many diseases such as allergies, asthma, gluten and gliadin intolerance, digestive disturbances, yeast infections, various mucous and congestive conditions, and several types of arthritis. Most grains are harvested and kept in storage, giving them the chance to begin the fermentation process and, therefore, most are filled with mold and fungus and have a high amount of mycrotoxins."

Reaching an Ecological Balance

Oils:
Oils are not really part of the Living Foods Lifestyle mainly because the processing used to get the concentrated oils from the source causes a loss of the natural balance. Nature intuitively knows how to put all the ingredients together in the perfect combination for the human body. When we manipulate foods in this manor, the body no longer recognizes it and does not know how to break down from this toxic form.

To get the oils our bodies need, use oily seeds and nuts even though they are difficult to digest and are very acid and mucus forming when not properly soaked. Soaked and sprouted seeds are much easier to digest, the enzyme inhibitors are released and the vitamin and mineral content is increased. The Ann Wigmore Institute uses a select few seeds and nuts (listed below) and always prepares them as milk, seed yogurt, seed cheese or a blended pâté. These seeds and nuts are the safest for Candida sufferers but also we feel confident that these truly are raw and not even mildly processed. They also have a much lower possibility of becoming rancid.

- Almonds
- Flaxseed
- Pumpkin Seed
- Sunflower Seed

Almonds must be used with caution as the United States has implemented pasteurization requirements. Organic raw almonds can still be purchased through local farmers markets as they are still allowed to sell raw almonds.

Ocean Vegetables:
Raw ocean vegetables are extremely rich in minerals. It is important to get them raw and organic to ensure the full benefit of the abundance of nutrients sea vegetables provide. At the Ann Wigmore Institute we use Nori, Dulse

and Kelp, but you could use other types such as Arame or Wakame.

Teas are not a Living Food therefore not part of my personal diet nor are they served at the Ann Wigmore Institute. However; Dr. Ann would warm water and soak grated ginger in it to prepare ginger water. Lemon and stevia could also be added to the ginger "tea" drink. If you choose to drink tea other safe mixtures for people with Candida include Burdock Root, Dandelion, Echinacea, Mathake, and Pau D' Arco.

Fungus Forming Foods to Avoid:

- Barley
- Cashews
- Corn
- Oats
- Peanuts
- Wheat
- Yeast

According to Dr Gabriel Cousens in his book Rainbow Green Live-Food Cuisine pg 25 "These foods have high mycrotoxin and fungal count and should be avoided." Other items he strongly recommends avoiding are listed in more detail in his book on page 26, briefly they are:

- **Alcohol** should be avoided for many reasons but primarily because it can convert back into acid aldehyde which is very acidic to the entire body but dangerously toxic to the liver
- **Soy sauce** (including nama shoyu) is another food high in micro-toxic fungi
- **Coffee and caffeine** are acidic and create acidification of the tissues
- **Tobacco** when cured or fermented has very high levels of yeast, fungus, and micro-toxins

Reaching an Ecological Balance

There is another important factor that we need to take in careful consideration and it is the fat levels in our diets. In my personal experience, I removed all the fat for eight days and slowly incorporated flaxseed, and then gradually I added other fats into my diet. In the Living Foods Lifestyle we are not too worried about the fats because we eat such a small quantity and limited variety of nuts, seeds and avocados. We basically use the varieties that we feel are the safest in terms of freshness and which also have the lowest mold content possibility.

Lalita's Personal Struggle

I used to be a typical Argentinean woman, enjoying family gatherings with the traditional barbecued meat as the main food attraction. My father loved to bring each child the first and "best" pieces of meat. He would lovingly place the first pieces of meat in our mouths before the rest of the meal was ready. From a very early age, meat and love went together, it was like the precious meat we were being so tenderly served was replacing the security and love an infant feels receiving his mother's milk.

At the age of 23 I graduated from the Universidad de Cuyo, Argentina as a Pharmacist. It was shortly after graduation that I had my first introduction to vegetarianism, which at the time was such a foreign concept for me to grasp. To me it was something crazy and difficult to understand, but for some reason I kept this vegetarian information stored in my memory bank. My first unsuccessful attempt at becoming a vegetarian came two years later. It was such a painful experience for me missing out on the family barbecue with my parents and siblings that I did not truly convert to an "established vegetarian" until the age of 38 (1986). Even then it was still painful not to be sharing the traditional barbecued meat with my family and even harder to explain my diet choice to them, but somehow I survived in my new vegetarian world. Nine months later my husband became a vegetarian, then one of my daughters, and later on my son. Some years later, my son married a vegetarian woman. They remain vegetarians, along with their children. It seems that each generation improves a little as the world becomes more educated about health.

Lalita's Personal Struggle

I was a vegetarian but I was a lacto-ova vegetarian (eating dairy and egg products), I had improved my diet substantially, but I kept eating fungi promoting foods that were creating a serious unbalance within my body.

In 1983 I developed a fungus in the nail of my left index finger but I did not make the connection that my lifestyle had anything to do with my fungus. This condition was upsetting to me because I loved my nails and had always been very proud of them. I decided to visit a doctor. I really believed that the doctor would take care of me, I was sure that he would give me some type of medication that would take care of that awful fungus. I had a big disappointment with that visit because after the doctor looked at my nails he said with a strong and convincing voice, "This condition is very difficult, almost impossible to eradicate, there is no medication for this condition." I was devastated; all I could think of was that I would have to live with this fungus for the rest of my life. I thought I had no other choice, so I went home in tears and forced myself to learn to live with this fungus. I accomplished this by trying not to pay too much attention to it and even denying to myself that I had this condition in my nail.

The next year we moved to New York; I was walking in a park in upstate New York when I saw a sign for a doctor that specialized in toenail and fingernail conditions including fungi! I was so excited, thinking that because I found a specialist, he would give me the illusive magic medicine to heal my condition. I made an appointment for the very next day. The specialist did pay more attention to my problem, looking carefully at my nail and finally deciding that I needed three treatments of an anti fungal medication injected under the nail. Along with this he gave

Lalita's Personal Struggle

me medication to take orally. I followed every instruction with such faith, certain that finally I would conquer and eradicate this ugly fungus. Needless to say the treatments did not work and in less than one month, the fungus spread into all but two of my nails. Sadly, these two nails served as a constant reminder that I once had beautiful hands. About this time in my life I moved into a more conscious vegetarian diet (honey instead of white sugar, whole wheat flour instead of white flour), although I still did not connect my fungus condition with my food choices. I had no clue that I would have to change my diet to get better. I learned to live with the fungus which had spread to most of my fingernails and shortly after it also started invading my toenails.

It was about 1985 and my youngest daughter had an ear infection that lasted for over two months. I faithfully kept bringing her to the pediatrician with the assurance that he would cure her with his "magic medicine". I was so afraid that if I did not follow the doctor's advice something terrible would happen to my daughter. I was taking her to the doctor every 15 days hoping each time that she would improve. The doctor became concerned that my daughter would lose her hearing. I talked to many other mothers and to the teachers from my daughter's pre-school about her chronic condition. The teachers advised me to discontinue the antibiotics and recommended that instead I put a clove of garlic in my daughter's ears every night. At first it sounded a little crazy to me, but I was willing to try almost anything so I interrupted the medication and started her on the garlic clove treatment. The next trip to the doctor's office confirmed that my daughter's chronic ear infection was finally gone, I could hardly believe it! This was a turning point for me, it was as though a light went on inside my head and I began to wake up. Slowly I started taking more and more steps to change my lifestyle. I began sharing yoga with my friends. All of us were embracing the idea that we needed to change our food but still I did not remove the fungus promoting foods because I did not know or understand the relationship between the fungus and my food choices. When I took yoga instructor training, I noticed that the fungus in my nails was improving. I lost one toenail, and a new nail started growing without fungus! I was so happy; I had new hopes for the end of this terrible invasion my body was experiencing. But I had many questions; I was not sure what was doing the healing. Was it the yoga? Was it because we were fasting with mostly water and a little rice? Again, I had no inkling of what was happening in my own body.

During this time I met a lady who was very tired and weak. We became friends and I remember she was so sick that she was not even able to drive her car. She told me that she had Candida. I did not understand or have any previous knowledge about this rare condition that according to her could invade the body. She asked me to prepare a special soup for her because of this condition and I did. Now that I understand so much more about the relationship between food and Candida, I realize why she could not improve from this condition even though she changed her diet. She had not given up the starchy vegetables like sweet potatoes, and hardly anything in her diet was living. The situation with my new friend and her strange condition was so foreign to me that I was thinking, "She is a sweet woman but she must have a mental condition." I truly felt this way because all that talk about Candida invading the body was such a strange concept to me, I just could not comprehend it at the time.

Lalita's Personal Struggle

For most of us it is difficult to realize that food, one of our main sources of comfort, a connection with our parents, our traditions, our very roots could possibly ever hurt us. The food that our mother's gave to us, how could that hurt us? Mom, such an important figure, Mom who knows what is best for us, Mom, our main support when we were so little and innocent, Mom who loved us and taught us what and how to eat. How could we believe these people with their crazy ideas and crazy books trying to tell us that Mom's food is wrong and making us sick? How can we reject such an important part of who we are?

I always felt that food was part of my identity and if I rejected the food that was part of who I was then I would be destroying part of myself. If most people feel this way, it is no wonder so many are dying prematurely with so many diseases. People have such a difficult time changing their diets for health reasons. It is so hard to understand that the main cause of the composting and recycling process our bodies go through trying to remove disease from itself is a direct result of poor food choices.

In 1990 we moved to Puerto Rico, I had to say good bye to my dear friends from New York who had all been such an inspiration and support system for me. They had faith in me and I in them; they knew about my nails and my concerns and loved me in spite of my insecurities and my condition. I knew it would be lonely without my support group.

We arrived in·P.R. on July 27, 1990. I did not know it at the time, but the "Mission" was waiting for me. I had given up my pharmaceutical career and was teaching yoga in P.R.

Lalita's Personal Struggle

About a year after relocating I accepted a job substitute teaching for the yoga instructor at the Ann Wigmore Institute. On July 4th, 1991, I arrived at the institute and Dr. Ann Wigmore was the first person I saw that early morning. My heart was beating like a bird that wanted to fly out of its cage. I could not understand these feelings but felt like a teenager on her first date, I was simply shaking with excitement. It was a historical day for me and for her too I guess because I became her disciple and now almost two decades later, my dearest friend and advocate, Leola Brooks and I, still share the Living Foods Lifestyle with all the students that come to learn how to take responsibility for their own health.

In that first meeting, my wisdom, the part of me that knows everything, instinctively said to me "You have arrived home." One time Dr. Ann said to me, "Lalita, your blood family is not the only family that you have, they are a part of your family, but your family is the whole world." When I became part of the Ann Wigmore Institute family, I became more in touch with my inner self, more in tune with the needs of my body, and with the needs of others. The doors were opening up to me and the world was becoming my family.

By this time the fungus was quite evident under and over my nails. My knees were dry, peeling and itching. I never suffered with a lack of energy like many people with Candida, but I had other symptoms such as muscle aches and a sore throat when I woke up in the morning, bloating, rectal itching, bad breath, dry mouth and frequently I had a sensation in my throat, coming from my chest that I was not able to breathe. I did not realize at the time that all these symptoms were related to the disease called

Lalita's Personal Struggle

Candida. The same disease my old friend from New York tried to explain to me years before that I could not understand. However, I did begin to notice that there was a connection between the symptoms and the amount of sweets that I ate.

I did not understand my Candida right away, it took me time to realize or accept what it was. During my first two years at the Institute I was dealing with my personal resistance to Living Foods. Remember, I was lacto–ova vegetarian so the transition to Living Foods was a huge adjustment for me. I was using large amounts of mangos to disguise the energy soup because the soup was a food that I was not able to connect with at all. I needed to cover the taste of the greens so I was eating more fruit than ever before, along with lots of nuts, seeds, coconut meat, and dehydrated foods. I was trying to replace breads, eggs, cheese, and milk yogurt with living substitutions. I was looking for animal protein. I was looking for bread, cookies, cakes, and ice cream; I was looking for all my old comfort foods. Then one day when I was feeling kind of crazy for food, I asked myself, "Do you really want to be in this lifestyle? Nobody is pushing you. You have a choice." I spent a few days thinking about this and realized that the motivation was coming from inside of me, from a place that I could not understand. I was looking for foods that would help me reach a higher level of meditation and this is the lifestyle that the Universe put in front of me. I was not balancing Living Foods in the beginning I was running away as much as I could from blended greens. As I was going through this process my situation with Candida continued to worsen and finally I started to pay attention to the warning signals my body was giving me.

Lalita's Personal Struggle

As the years went by, students came with more and more concerns related to Candida, I began to study and learn more about this ecologically unbalancing condition. I started sharing with the students everything I was learning about Candida. Some students were aware of Candida and others simply went to my new class out of curiosity. The latter would look at me like I was talking in another language, it seemed to be so strange for them and they could not believe that they could have an overgrowth of this fungus called Candida.

I tried so many ways to work with my own Candida. Energy soup without the fruit, but keeping the fat, then energy soup without the fat but keeping the fruit (the best for me because I love fruit) then finally energy soup with only dulse, lemon and ginger. Then I incorporated more and more sauerkraut, this combined with the energy soup was my personal healing path. I was also inspired by Gabriel Cousens, M.D. and his clinical studies on his own staff adopting a low–glycemic (low-sweet) diet, and then voluntarily continuing on the maintenance phase to this day.

I feel great walking into my 60's with the realization that I have to eat less food to be healthy. Mostly I eat low glycemic food, primarily energy soup, sauerkraut and wheat grass juice. I also cleansed my body for two weeks with only energy soup, wheatgrass juice and water, then I added sauerkraut, flax seed cream and low glycemic fruit about once a week. Candida has been a long time special guest in my body that I owe the principle of moderation with everything I feed it. Intellectually I knew about moderation for a long time before I practiced it. Candida has shown me very clearly that every action has a reaction and that everything I eat or drink will have a positive or negative effect. Looking back I can categorize myself as a compulsive eater and very attached to sweets. From a very early age my parents, like many other parents, rewarded me with chocolate, cookies, candies and other sweets. No wonder it was such a struggle to break this cycle of unconsciously binging on sweets.

For so many years my poor colon was crying for Lactobacillus to come and do their balancing job inside me but I never gave my body the nourishment it needed to completely heal itself. During my Candida journey I learned that eating without control, especially sweets and fats; really hurt me both physically and emotionally. It took me time to get it but when I finally did understand and accept it, I was able to conquer the Candida overgrowth. Only then could Candida again become a regular part of my micro-ecological system without the need to reproduce like crazy trying desperately to recycle me. The environment within my body no longer pushes Candida into over reproduction because I am finally in tune with the needs of my body and in turn, my body is in tune with nature.

Candida was not an easy journey for me because at first I did not understand or believe in it and later I just did not understand exactly how to conquer it. The more research I did and the more people I talked to about it, the more I began to understand Candida. Clearly, the more in tune I became with my own body, the better equipped I was to give my body the fuel it needed to balance itself.
As the years passed, my friend Candida slowly became more evident to me. Today I consider my Candida in remission. I fully understand the need to have balance in

my life and how closely related this balance is to everything I put in my mouth. Like many people, I had a tendency to overeat when I was feeling the least bit of stress in my life. I would overeat with sweet fruits, dates, nuts and other types of fats. I feel fortunate that I have developed such a keen sensitivity to these types of foods; I believe this sensitivity was my gift from my years with Candida. Even today if I overeat sweets or fats my body reacts leaving me feeling sluggish and tired. This sensitivity is a constant reminder to me of the need for living a life filled with balance and moderation so I can enjoy the good health and abundant energy I have grown accustomed to.

Lalita's Personal Struggle

Leola said that Candida is an elusive thing, and society as a whole is just beginning to open up to this Candida subject. I was talking about my nails with close friends and family but I was in denial that I had an imbalance or that my symptoms were related to food. It is very strange to think back that in the beginning I was not doing Living Foods because of my nails, I was doing Living Foods primarily to heighten my meditation experience and secondarily because I wanted to prevent future health problems. We humans can be so confused about our own bodies and what they are trying to tell us. As I learn more and more how to read my own body signals, I am developing a deep-rooted compassion for myself and for others that are entrapped in some level of a misunderstood recycling process.

May this book help you find the path to success for restoring the ecological balance within your own body.

Food Sources

We are slowly destroying the ecological balance of our planet by adding chemicals to our crops.
When the planet is destroyed, what will happen to us?
–Lalita Salas

Organic: Whenever possible use fresh pesticide free organic ingredients. Pesticides are a poison designed to kill living organisms and can be very harmful to humans.

Water: Always use a pure source of water such as filtered or reverse osmosis water. Distilled water can be used if you prefer, but prior to use put a few blades of wheatgrass in the water and allow it to stand in the sun for ½ hour. Ann Wigmore (and many Living Food resources) consider distilled water "dead water" but the blade of wheatgrass and sunshine will bring some life back into the water.

Nuts, Seeds and Grains: must be properly prepared. This recipe book assumes all nuts are soaked for the appropriate time and all seeds and grains are soaked and sprouted. The only nuts we feel safe to use for Candida are raw almonds which must be soaked and peeled for most recipes. Among the approved seed list are un-hulled flax seed, pumpkin seeds and sunflower seeds. Approved grains include buckwheat, quinoa, amaranth and millet. It is always important to blend nuts and seeds very well to produce a consistency that is easier to digest. Please refer to the sprouting section on page 107.

Food Sources

Onions and Garlic: Ann Wigmore preferred chives over other types of onions because they are mainly greens and milder than the others. The only onions we use are scallions and then only the green portion. Onions and garlic have medicinal properties and should not be used like an ordinary food source.

Celery Powder: In the recipes that call for celery powder it can be considered an optional ingredient and can be substituted with dulse. If you purchase dehydrated and ground celery make sure it is pure organic celery and contains nothing else in the ingredient list. To make your own "salt" dice up 3-4 packages of celery and dehydrate at 105F for 12-15 hours. Grind the dehydrated celery in a dry blender or coffee grinder. This will yield about 1 ounce of salt or powder.

Ground Ingredients: In recipes calling for ground ingredients such as flax seed, quinoa, buckwheat or sunflower the preparation is the same for soaking and sprouting. (See the sprouting section on page 107.) When the seeds have been soaked and sprouted, spread on mesh dehydrator sheets and dehydrate at 105F for approximately 12 hours. Using a coffee grinder or dry blender; grind the seeds into a powdery consistency.

Sauerkraut: For recipes calling for sauerkraut see the cultured foods section on page 95.

Living Foods

This guide for Candida health restoration is based on Living Foods. Living Foods are the key to maintaining or restoring your body to ultimate health. Living Foods are an enzyme rich food source which is the key to restoring and strengthening a weakened immune system.

At the Ann Wigmore Natural Health Institute in Puerto Rico we teach the complete Living Foods Lifestyle, but this book focuses mainly on the Living Foods part of the lifestyle with the primary focus on restoring the ecological balance so your body can eliminate the overgrowth of Candida yeast. There are many antifungal prescriptions on the market but based on my personal experience I believe it is possible to conquer Candida with the food we eat.

Living Foods are the purest form of nourishment your body can receive. They are fresh organically grown foods prepared in a way that is easy-to-digest nourishment allowing easier assimilation of the vast vitamins and minerals in these foods. Living Foods contain every nutrient and vital element your body needs, they support the body's cleansing process and help to eliminate strong cravings and also help us overcome other food addictions. Most living foods are loaded with a healthy source of natural fiber that our body needs to help with internal cleansing.

Living Foods

Key Methods with Living Foods

- Soaking and Sprouting – Nuts, Seeds, & Grains
  - Releases enzyme inhibitors
  - Increase vitamins & minerals
  - Produces a more alkaline forming food source
  - Offers a much less mucus forming diet
  - Provides easier to digest nourishment
  - Nourishment is easily assimilated into the body and the protein is a higher quality food, which is low in fat and cholesterol free

- Blending
  - Easier for the body to digest
  - Easier for the body to assimilate the nourishment
  - Provides a natural concentrated nourishment

- Culturing or Fermenting
  - Helps restore friendly bacteria (lactobacilli)
  - Hard to digest foods become easier to digest
    - Cabbage
    - Carrots
    - Broccoli
    - Cauliflower

With all of our key methods you will notice the emphasis put on "easy-to-digest" nourishment. Many people wonder why it is so important to prepare these foods so they become easier to digest. For example why would we blend our food? That is not natural. The truth of the matter is that most people's digestive systems are not at their peak vitality. Our digestive systems have been weakened through years of eating de-naturalized, processed, and unbalanced cooked foods. That is why it is very important to give our digestive systems every advantage that we can with our food preparation.

Living Foods

You will also notice that we use very few seasonings or spices in our food preparation. Seasonings can distract us from the natural flavor of the food we are eating confusing our taste buds in the process. In addition, and this is a major issue, seasoning often causes us to lose a sense of "how much is enough" when we are eating. In many circumstances this results in eating more than the body can handle for successful digestion and assimilation.

Many people no longer eat for health and nutrition; many eat simply as a form of entertainment or comfort. The body | food connection tends to get lost over the years and the body can no longer easily identify specific vitamins and minerals and becomes confused with how to process these un-natural foods. When this happens we have upset the natural balance within ourselves and are at a complete disconnect with nature.

The Living Foods Lifestyle (LFL) supports our body's natural cleansing and detoxifying process. It also helps eliminate strong cravings and aids in overcoming food addictions.

The LFL balances us physically, mentally, emotionally and spiritually.

"It is time for you to nurture your body and give it the tools it needs to restore the ecological balance it deserves."
–Lalita Salas

Breakfast

Start your day with an enzyme rich nutritional living breakfast.

Amaranth Creamy Cereal

1 cup amaranth, sprouted
1 cup strawberries
½ cup sunflower milk
5-6 stevia leaves or green stevia powder to taste

Place all ingredients in a blender and blend enough to get a creamy, smooth mixture.

Yields 2 servings

You can substitute the strawberries with blueberries or any other berry.

The sunflower milk can be replaced with almond or pumpkin milk.

See the recipe for seed milk in the milk section on page 93.

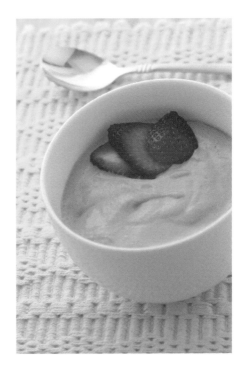

Breakfast

Berry Flake Cereal

2 cups strawberries or blueberries
10 – 30 stevia leaves
1 cup flax seed, soaked and ground

Blend the berries with the stevia, mix in a bowl with the flax seed, spread on the dehydrator sheets to a very thin consistency and cut into ½ inch bite size squares. Dehydrate for approximately 12 hours

Serve with sunflower or almond milk. This cereal can be served with fresh blueberries or strawberries.

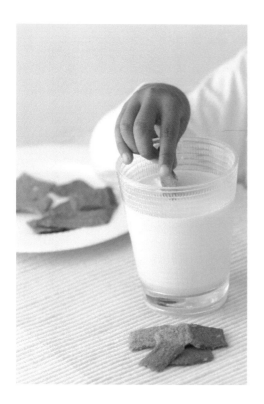

This recipe can be used as a cereal or as cookies.

To get the cookie consistency as shown here simply spread the mixture on the dehydrator sheets to a slightly thicker consistency.

Yields 2 servings

Breakfast

Breakfast Smoothie

1 medium apple
2 cups fresh or frozen strawberries or blueberries
8 oz of baby spinach
¼ - ½ cup filtered water or rejuvelac

Blend the apples and berries until a creamy consistency is reached. Add the spinach and blend until smooth. If you do not get a smooth creamy consistency when blending the apples and berries add ¼ - ½ cup of filtered water or rejuvelac. Pour the smoothie into glasses and garnish with fresh berries.

Yields 2 servings

Remember, the greens should have the least amount of blending time as possible so always add them as your last ingredient. The spinach can be replaced with your favorite greens however, make sure the greens are not too bitter.

If you are having problems getting your family to eat their greens, smoothies are a great way to incorporate more greens into their diets. Although listed as a breakfast choice, Smoothies can be served any time of day as a meal or a snack.

Breakfast

Living Quinoa Cereal

1 cup quinoa; sprouted, dehydrated and ground
1 cup sunflower milk
1 teaspoon lemon juice
5-6 fresh stevia leaves, chopped or green stevia powder to taste

Combine the above ingredients in a cereal bowl, mix and serve. Optionally you can serve this dish garnished with fresh berries. This is one of my favorite cereals. Refer to the milk section on page 93 for directions for seed and almond milk.

Yields 1 serving

"For much of my life I had incurable health problems, but slowly I learned that there is nothing that nature, if given a chance, can not overcome." **–Dr. Ann Wigmore**

Breakfast

Buckwheat Apple Cereal

1 cup Buckwheat grouts, sprouted
1 cup almond milk
1 cup apple
5-6 stevia leaves or green stevia powder to taste

Place all ingredients in a blender and blend just enough to get a creamy smooth texture. Serve in a cereal bowl. See the milk section on page 93 for the directions to make almond milk.

Optionally you can garnish this dish with apples.

Yields 2 servings

Appetizers & Side Dishes

Any of the appetizers and/or side dishes can be served with fresh vegetable sticks, or with any of the chips or crackers in the crackers, chips and bread section. Or my personal favorite is over a bed of greens.

Almond Sauce

1 teaspoon chives or scallions, chopped
1 teaspoon celery powder or dulse (optional)
1 teaspoon lemon juice
$2/3$ cup water
1 cup almonds, soaked and peeled

Mix and blend the first four ingredients, when well blended add the almonds and blend until you get a smooth creamy sauce.

Yields 1 ½ cups

See the Sprouting section on page 107 for directions on soaking and peeling almonds.

Basic Pumpkin Seed Pâté

½ cup pumpkin seeds, sprouted
1 teaspoon cilantro, chopped
1 teaspoon celery powder or dulse (optional)
1 teaspoon lemon juice

Blend all the ingredients and serve.
Yields ½ cup

Blended Salsa

1 dehydrated tomato
1 tomato, chopped
1 carrot, chopped
¼ cup cilantro, chopped
½ cup chives or scallions, chopped
1 teaspoon lemon juice
1 teaspoon celery powder or dulse (optional)

Soak the dehydrated tomato in pure water for 1 hour or until the desired consistency is reached. Blend all the ingredients and serve.

Yields 1 cup

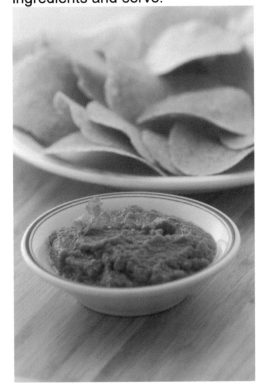

Guacamole

2 medium avocados
⅓ cup chives or scallions, chopped
1 small tomato, diced
1 zucchini, diced
⅓ cup red bell pepper, diced
1 teaspoon lemon juice
½ cup celery, diced
1 teaspoon celery powder or dulse (optional)

Mash or cube the avocados and mix with the other ingredients.

Yields 2 ½ cups

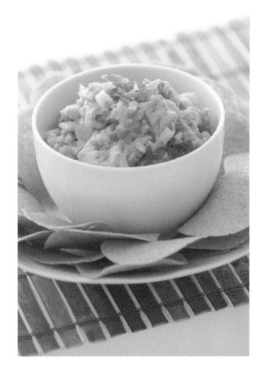

Zucchini Hummus

I was inspired for this recipe by a creation of Dr.'s Rick and
Karen Dina.

1 medium zucchini, chopped
2 teaspoon lemon juice
1 teaspoon celery powder or dulse (optional)
2 teaspoon flax seed, soaked
¼ cup almonds, soaked and peeled

Blend the first three ingredients until smooth, then add the
flax seed and almonds and continue blending until you get
a creamy mixture.
Yields 1 ½ cups

See page 108 for
directions on soaking
and peeling almonds.

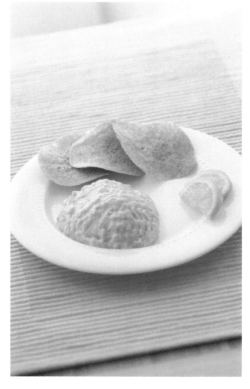

Soups

Cucumber Soup

1 medium cucumber, grated
2 cups seed milk (pumpkin or sunflower)
1 apple
1 tablespoon kelp
8 -12 cucumber slices
2 tablespoon chives or scallions, diced

Blend the apple and seed milk. Combine with grated cucumber. Serve in individual bowls decorated with cucumber slices and chives. Sprinkle with kelp.

Yields 2 servings

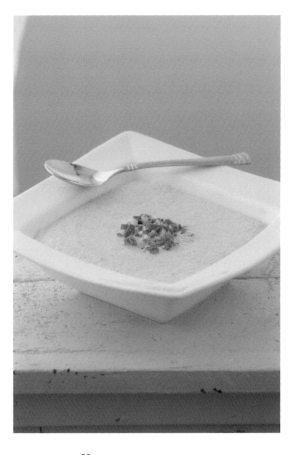

For a seed milk recipe see the milk section on page 93.

Salads

Energy Soup

Energy soup is a complete food that is rich in fiber and contains an abundance of nutrients in a balanced form. It is easy-to-digest nourishment and filled with alkaline forming minerals making this one of the most valuable foods in the Living Foods Lifestyle. Energy soup is a complete food with the combination of fiber and nutrients thus allowing your body to cleanse and rebuild at the same time.

1 ½ cups zucchini or 1 cup of zucchini and ½ cup of carrots
⅛ cup lentil sprouts or pea sprouts
1 tablespoon of leafy dulse or
1 teaspoon of granulated dulse
½ cup Rejuvelac or pure water
14 cups sunflower greens
6 cups buckwheat greens
1 medium avocado or ½ cup seed yogurt

Blending Steps
Mix the zucchini, carrots, and sprouts with the Rejuvelac and blend well.

Add the avocado and blend lightly.

Add the greens and dulse, blending and pushing the greens down all the time to facilitate the quickest blending time. This will help prevent the soup from becoming bitter.

Yields 2 quarts

Salads

*note: The sunflower and buckwheat could be replaced with a mix of many other greens such as collard greens (remove stack), kale greens, cilantro, watercress, parsley, celery greens, napa cabbage, bok choy , dark leaf lettuce, alfalfa or clover sprouts, swiss chard leaves (remove stack), cactus pads, edible weeds: purslane, lamb's quarters, young dandelion, etc.

.

Use strong tasting greens sparingly as their flavor will overpower the taste of the soup. An example of a very strong green is watercress or arugula.

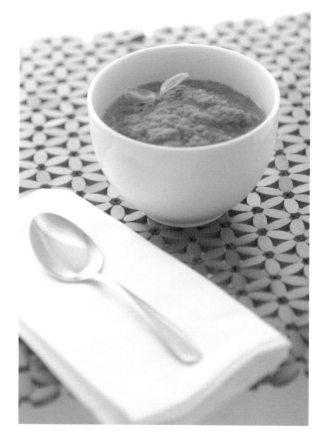

Salads

Celery Soup

2 apples
1 small bunch of celery (including greens)
2 tablespoon parsley
1 small avocado
2 cups sunflower greens
2 small zucchini

Blend all ingredients until you reach a smooth creamy texture.

Yields 2–4 servings

"I remember my addiction to candy…. I had to learn the importance of not feeling defeated after making a big mistake…. I had to learn how to accept myself and to let go of my guilt and powerlessness. After I accomplished this, I was free to move on while being open to from the next challenge or opportunity."
–Dr. Ann Wigmore; Rebuild Your Health

Salads

Avocado Chowder

1 small avocado, diced
½ cup grated carrots
½ cup grated red pepper
½ cup grated celery
1 cup chopped chives or scallions
1 tablespoon kelp or leafy dulse
2 tablespoons sauerkraut
Lemon Juice to taste (optional)

Yields 2-3 servings

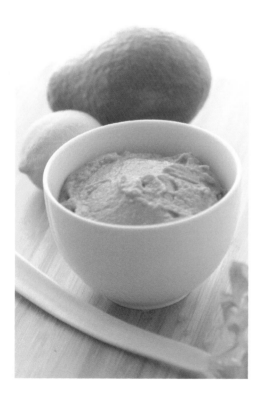

Blend the avocado until creamy. Add the remaining ingredients and blend very briefly to keep the thick chowdery consistency. Add the sauerkraut and mix by hand.

See the cultured foods section on page 95 for the sauerkraut recipe.

Salads

Vegetable Soup

1 carrot
2-3 spinach or chard leaves
½ small cucumber
1 cup chives or scallions
2-3 napa cabbage or collard green leaves
1 medium tomato
½ cup Rejuvelac or pure water
1 tablespoon celery powder or dulse (optional)

Blend all ingredients until smooth and creamy. Serve in individual bowls and garnish with grated carrots or red pepper.

Yields 1-2 servings

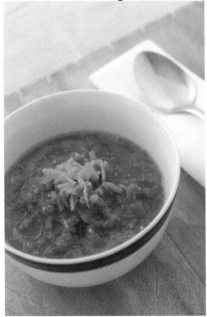

To thicken any vegetable soup, blend in an avocado or sprouted sunflower seeds.

Salads

Avocado Sprout Salad

1 medium avocado
2 ½ cups alfalfa or clover sprouts
½ cup celery, diced
½ cup chives, diced
½ cup carrots, sliced
1 cup red pepper, diced
3 tablespoons lemon juice
3 tablespoons celery powder or dulse (optional)

In a glass mixing bowl, combine all ingredients and mix well.

Yields 2-3 servings

Simple Healthy Salad

1 cup sunflower or buckwheat greens
1 cup alfalfa or fenugreek sprouts
Slices of zucchini and red pepper
Juice of ½ lemon

In a large salad bowl mix the greens and sprouts. Decorate with the zucchini and red pepper, sprinkle with lemon juice and serve.

Yields 2 servings

"It is your birthright to be healthy." **–Dr. Ann Wigmore**

Salads

It's not the food in your life that will bring you ultimate health; it's the life in your food. **–Michele Jarvey**

Creamy Cucumber Salad

2 cucumbers, sliced very thin
½ cup sunflower or pumpkin seed yogurt
Juice of ½ lemon
Celery powder or dulse to taste (optional)
⅓ cup clover sprouts
⅓ cup alfalfa sprouts
⅓ cup broccoli sprouts

Toss the cucumber slices with the yogurt and lemon. Sprinkle with celery powder or dulse. Serve over the bed of mixed sprouts.

Yields 2 servings

Rhio's Cucumbers & Cream Salad in her book Hooked on Raw inspired me to create this healthy and delicious salad.

Salads

Tabouli Salad

½ cup quinoa, sprouted
1 cup parsley, finely chopped
¼ cup cucumber, seeded and finely chopped
⅛ cup red pepper, finely diced
⅛ cup yellow pepper, finely diced
1 tablespoon lemon juice
1 tablespoon celery powder or dulse (optional)
1 cup carrot juice

Combine the first 7 ingredients in a mixing bowl and marinate for one hour. Add the carrot juice, toss the salad and marinate for an additional ½ hour.

Yields 2 servings

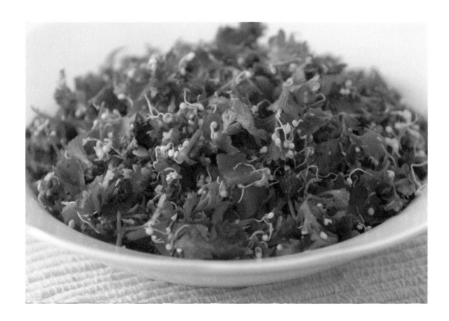

Salads

Tossed Green Salad

1 cup romaine lettuce
1 cup sunflower greens
¼ cup parsley, finely chopped
¼ cup watercress leaves or baby greens
½ cup nut milk
¼ cup chives or scallions, diced
Juice of ½ lemon

Cut the greens into bite sized pieces and put in a bowl, add the parsley, chives and watercress or baby greens. Pour lemon juice over the greens so that each leaf is well coated. Sprinkle with the nut milk and serve.

Yields 2 servings

"There are many antifungal prescriptions on the market but based on my personal experience I believe it is possible to conquer Candida with the food we eat."
–Lalita Salas

Entrées

The beauty and simplicity of these dishes will delight even your cooked food guests.

Zucchini Spaghetti

2 small zucchini
3 teaspoon celery powder or dulse (optional)
¼ cup lemon juice

With a spiral vegetable slicer grate the zucchini into spaghetti. After grating, cut the pasta into reasonable lengths. This makes it easier to toss and eat.

In a small bowl, mix the celery powder with the lemon juice. Toss the spaghetti with the lemon mix; let stand overnight in the refrigerator.

Serve with Marinara or Carrot sauce and sprinkled with Parmesan Cheese. See the sauces and dressings section on page 87.

Yields 2 servings

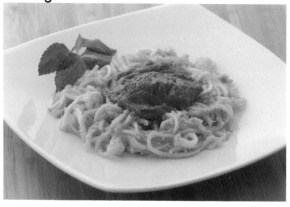

Entrées

Almond Pâté

4 cups almonds, soaked and peeled
1 cup carrots, chopped
2 cups buckwheat greens
2 cups purslane
1 cup celery leaves, chopped
1 cup parsley, chopped
¼ cup oregano, chopped
¾ cup chives or scallions or chives
½ cup basil, chopped
⅓ cup leafy dulse
¼ cup ginger
¼ cup rejuvelac
¼ cup lemon juice
⅓ cup orange or red pepper

Serves 10 – 15

With your omega or champion juicer using the blank plate, process only the almonds, the second time through the juicer alternate all of the ingredients except the soft greens. Repeat this process a third time passing everything through. Form the mixture into a loaf and place in a glass pan, cover with a cheese cloth and let process un-refrigerated for approximately 3 hours.

Serve the pâté with fresh vegetable sticks, on top of a bed of lettuce, or as stuffing in a tomato or red pepper.

Any of the greens for the almond pâté, can be replaced with substitute greens. For a different flavor altogether the almonds can be replaced with sunflower or pumpkin seeds.

Entrées

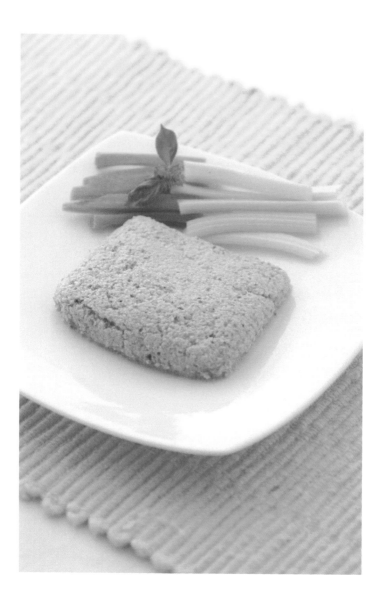

See the Sprouting section on page 107 for directions on soaking and peeling almonds.

Entrées

Pizza

Crust
½ cup Buckwheat grouts; sprouted, dehydrated, and ground
½ cup quinoa; sprouted, dehydrated, and ground
1 cup flax seed; soaked, dehydrated, and ground
1 tablespoon celery powder or dulse (optional)
½ cup carrot pulp
⅓ cup red pepper, diced
⅓ cup yellow pepper, diced
⅓ cup chives or scallions, chopped

Mix all ingredients and work with your hands until you have a well formed dough. When the dough is pliable form into individual size pizza crusts. Dehydrate the crusts at 115F for 4 hours on one side then flip the crust and dehydrate 4 more hours or until desired firmness is reached. It is easier to work with this dough if you wear gloves.

Yields 3 – 4 crusts

Entrées

Topping
Spread the crust with seed cheese, marinara or carrot sauce. Garnish with fresh diced vegetables and sprinkle with almond, sunflower or pumpkin parmesan cheese. See the parmesan cheese, marinara and carrot sauce recipes in the sauces and dressings section on page 87.

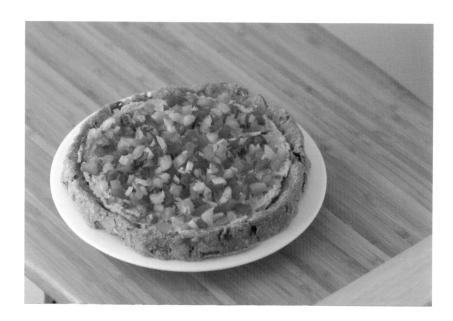

Entrées

Garden Burgers

½ cup sunflower seed; sprouted, dehydrated, and ground
¼ cup quinoa; sprouted and ground
½ cup carrot pulp or shredded carrot
2 tablespoons celery, finely chopped
2 tablespoons chives, finely chopped
2 tablespoons parsley, finely chopped
1 tablespoon red peppers, finely chopped
1 tablespoon yellow peppers, finely chopped
3 tablespoons flax seed, soaked and ground
3 tablespoons celery powder or dulse (optional)
6 tablespoons water (optional)

Put the first 8 ingredients into a medium-sized bowl and mix well. Add the remaining ingredients and work with your hands until you have a consistency that can be formed into patties.

Form into six patties approximately ½ inch thick. Place in the dehydrator at 115F for 4 hours. Flip the burgers and continue dehydrating for an additional 4 hours or until the desired consistency is reached.

Entrées

This dish is excellent served on a bed of fresh greens or with a side salad.

This is a great transitional food for people as well as a treat for seasoned raw fooders. I like to prepare this meal for guests that are still eating cooked foods as an introduction to living foods.

Yields 3 – 6 servings

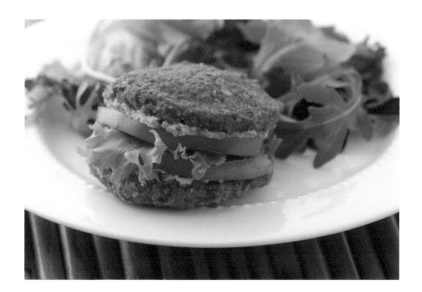

Entrées

Stuffed Avocados

1 avocado, halved and pitted
¼ cup sauerkraut or veggie-kraut
1 tablespoon lemon juice
1 tablespoon celery powder or dulse (optional)
⅛ cup sprouts

Mix the sauerkraut with the sprouts and celery powder.

Sprinkle the avocado with lemon juice, place 2 tablespoons of sauerkraut mix in each avocado half and sprinkle with dulse flakes.

Place on a bed of greens and serve. See the recipe for sauerkraut in the Cultured Foods section on page 95.

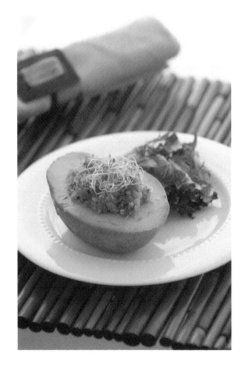

Yields 2 servings

Desserts

Almond Strawberry Cream

½ cup almonds, soaked and peeled
2 cups strawberries
15 stevia leaves (optional)
¼ cup water

Blend the almond
and water until
the almonds are
well broken. Add
the strawberries
and stevia;
continue blending
until a smooth
creamy texture is
reached.

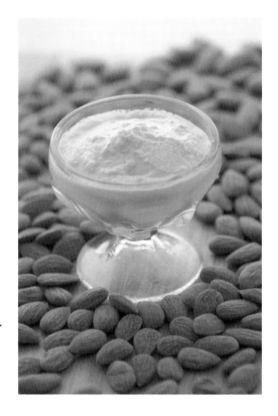

Yields 2 servings

This dish can be
served alone or
over fresh berries.

Refer to the Sprouting section on page 107 for directions
on soaking and peeling almonds.

Desserts

Apple Pie

Crust
½ cup sunflower seeds, soaked, dehydrated and ground
½ cup flax seed, soaked and ground
23 stevia leaves
¼ cup water

Blend the stevia with the water, transfer to a glass bowl and add the sunflower and flax seed and mix with your hands. Press the mixture into a glass 9-inch rectangular pan.

Apple Slices
3 apples, sliced in the Mandolin
1 tablespoon lemon juice
10 stevia leaves, blended
¼ cup water

Cut the apples in very thin slices and sprinkle with lemon juice. Blend the stevia and water and pour over the apples, soak for at least 15 minutes.

Filling
6 medium apples
½ tablespoon ginger, grated
½ cup flax seed, soaked and ground
10 stevia leaves

Process the apples, ginger and stevia in a food processor with the "S" blade or a blender. Put the mixture in a glass container and add the flax seed, mix very well.

Topping
5 medium Granny Smith apples
¼ cup water
½ tsp ginger, grated

10 stevia leaves
½ cup flax seed, soaked and ground

Blend the first 4 ingredients until smooth. Add the flax seed and blend until the seeds are well broken or until you get a smooth creamy consistency. Allow to stand in the refrigerator until you are ready to assemble the pie.

To Assemble the Pie

Put a layer of apple slices on the crust, followed by a layer of the filling. Keep layering in this way until you run out of ingredients. Cover with the topping and decorate with apple slices or ground sunflower seeds and sprinkle with cinnamon.

Yields 8-10 servings

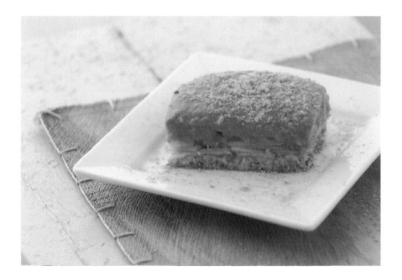

Desserts

Sunflower Cherry Cream

½ cup sunflower seeds, soaked and ground
2 cups cherries
⅓ cup water

Blend all the ingredients together until a smooth creamy texture is reached. This dish can be served alone or over fresh berries or cherries.

Yields 2 servings

Quinoa Raspberry Delight

2 cups raspberries
⅔ cup quinoa; sprouted, dehydrated, and ground
15 stevia leaves
⅓ cup water

Blend the raspberries with the water and stevia, pour the mixture into a bowl add the quinoa and mix until a creamy texture is reached.

Yields 2 servings

Living foods for a living body, that's where pure vitality comes from. –**Michele Jarvey**

Desserts

Avocado Strawberry Pudding

½ avocado
1 ½ cups strawberries
Stevia leaves to taste (optional)

Blend the strawberries with the stevia then add the avocado and blend until a smooth creamy texture is reached.

Yields 2 servings

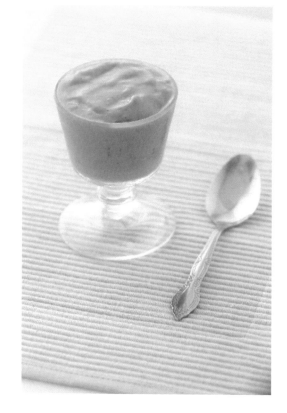

Crackers, Chips and Bread

With crackers and chips I sometimes make round chips by placing individual spoonful size servings on the dehydrator sheets and spreading to the desired consistency. Other times I spread the dough evenly across the dehydrator sheet and score into square or rectangular shapes when I flip the crackers. Raw crackers, chips and bread are very delicious and healthy replacement for "cooked" breads. These foods can be very important during your transitional period.

Zucchini Flax Crackers

4 medium zucchini peeled and diced
1 tomato
¼ cup fresh chopped dill
1 tablespoon celery powder or dulse (optional)
⅓ cup sunflower seeds, soaked and sprouted
1 cup flax seed, soaked and ground

Put first 5 ingredients in the blender and blend until a smooth consistency is reached. Pour mixture in a bowl and add the ground flax seed and mix well. Spoon the flax seed dough onto a mesh dehydrator sheet and dehydrate at 115F for 10 hours. Flip crackers and continue dehydrating for about 8 hours or until the desired texture is reached.

Yields 4-5 trays

Crackers, Chips and Bread

Buckwheat Flax Crackers

2 cups buckwheat grouts, sprouted
1 carrot
¼ cup chives or scallions, chopped
½ red bell pepper
1 ½ cups water
1 tomato
2 stalks of celery
1 cup flax seed, soaked and ground

Put first 7 ingredients in the blender and blend until smooth. Pour mixture into a bowl, add ground flax seed and mix well. Spoon the flax seed dough onto a mesh dehydrator sheet and dehydrate at 115F for 10 hours. Flip crackers and continue dehydrating for 8 hours or until the desired texture is reached.

Yields 4-6 trays

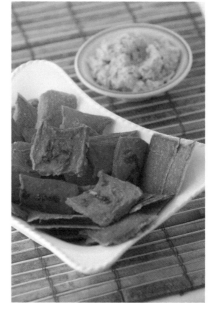

Crackers, Chips and Bread

Vegetable Flax Crackers

1 cup whole flax seed, soaked
⅓ cup flax seed, soaked and ground
2 cups water
2 carrots
1 tomato
8 stalks of celery
4 leaves fresh basil
½ cup scallions or chives, chopped

Blend all ingredients in a blender except the ground flax seed. In a large bowl, add the blended ingredients to the ground flax seed and mix with your hands.

Spoon the flax seed dough on a mesh dehydrator sheet and dehydrate at 115F for 10 hours. Flip crackers and continue dehydrating for 8 hours or until the desired texture is reached.

Yields 4-6 trays

The number of trays each recipe will yield will depend on how thick or thin you spread the dough.

Quinoa Chips

1 cup quinoa; sprouted, dehydrated, and ground
⅓ cup flax seed, soaked and ground
1 medium yellow pepper
2 stalks of celery
½ cup dehydrated tomato
½ cup chives or scallions
2 teaspoons cumin
1 teaspoon kelp
½ cup leafy dulse, soaked and cut into small pieces
(optional)
¼ cup water or lemon juice

Blend slightly the yellow pepper, celery, tomato, chives, cumin, and kelp with the lemon juice or water .In a mixing bowl, combine the ground quinoa and flax seed with the blended vegetables; mix well. Stir in the leafy dulse.

Spoon the dough onto a mesh dehydrator sheet spreading into a thin chip consistency. Dehydrate at 115F for 10 hours. Flip chips and continue dehydrating for an additional 8 hours or until the desired consistency is reached

Yields 4-6 trays

Crackers, Chips and Bread

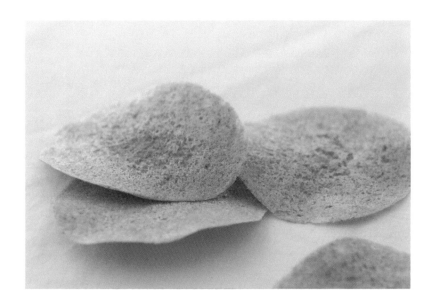

Crackers, Chips and Bread

Quinoa Flax Bread

4 cups quinoa; sprouted, dehydrated, and ground
2 cups flax seed, soaked and ground
1 cup chives or scallions, chopped
1 tablespoon celery powder or dulse (optional)
½ teaspoon kelp
¼ teaspoon cumin (optional)
2 orange peppers
2 red peppers
½ cup water

In a Vita-mix, blend the water, with the orange and red peppers and set aside.

In a large mixing bowl combine the flax seed and quinoa; add the chives and mix well. Add the celery powder, kelp, and cumin and mix well. Add the pepper mixture one cup at a time combining well with your hands into a doughy texture.

With wet hands, roll the dough into ½" by 5 rolls. Braid two rolls together squeezing the ends together. This process will allow for a more even distribution of heat allowing the center of the loaf to dehydrate well preventing a doughy middle and premature mold growth, or form into thin loaves as shown here.

Sprinkle the Teflex sheets with water and place the loaves on the Teflex sheets skipping every other shelf allowing room for the bread to rise an additional ½ inch. Dehydrator at 1"15F for 24 – 48 hours depending on the consistency you prefer.

Yields 4-6 loaves

Crackers, Chips and Bread

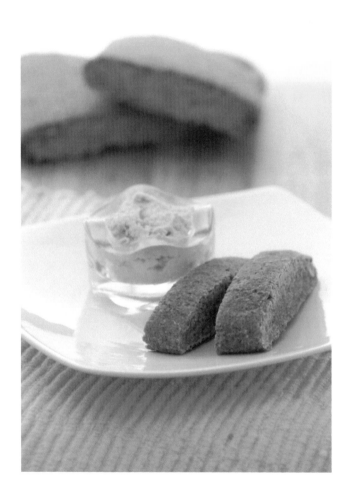

Sauces and Dressings

Marinara Sauce

¾ cup diced red pepper
2 cups Roma Tomatoes, chopped
1 cup dehydrated tomatoes
¼ cup basil, diced

Soak the dehydrated tomatoes, drain and blend with the fresh tomatoes and red pepper. Transfer to a serving bowl and mix in the basil.

Yields 3 cups

This sauce is good over zucchini spaghetti as shown, or as a dip for chips or veggie sticks. To use as a pizza sauce add 1 teaspoon of dried oregano.

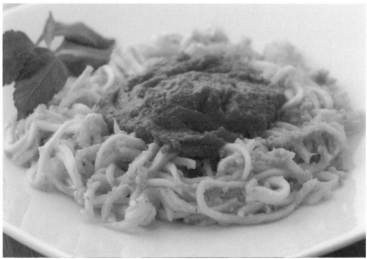

A friend and co-worker, Louise Dwyer, contributed the marinara sauce recipe.

Sauces and Dressings

Parmesan Cheese

1 cup of Almonds, Sunflower or Pumpkin

Soak and sprout the seeds. If you are using almonds, soak the almonds rinsing twice a day, if you are unable to rinse twice, soak the almonds in the refrigerator to prevent premature fermentation. Almonds must be soaked and peeled. Refer to the Sprouting section on page – for directions on soaking and peeling almonds.

Dehydrate the nuts or seeds at 115° for 12 - 24 hours or until dry. In a dry blender or coffee grinder, grind until a dried cheese consistency is reached.

Yields ¾ cup

Carrot Sauce

2 carrots
1 medium zucchini
½ cup chives or scallions
2 stalks of celery
⅛ cup red pepper
½ cup water
⅓ cup ginger juice
1 teaspoon celery powder or dulse (optional)

Yields approximately 1 cup

Blend all the ingredients together until you get a smooth texture. This is ideal on top of zucchini spaghetti or as a pizza sauce. It can be used on anything as a replacement of tomato sauce.

Tomatillo Sauce

½ cup tomatillo
1 teaspoon celery powder or dulse (optional)
¼ cup ginger, grated
1 tablespoon celery, chopped
15 stevia leaves or a pinch of green stevia powder

Blend all together.

Yields ½ cup

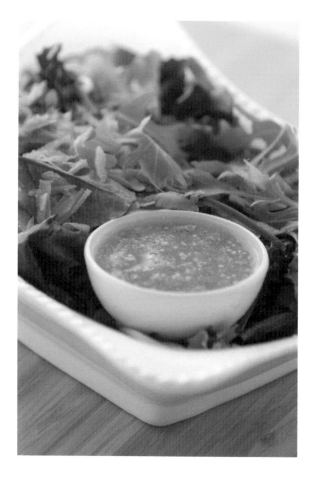

Apple Ginger Dressing

2 medium green apples
2 tablespoons lemon juice
¼ cup water
½ teaspoon ginger, grated

Blend all the ingredients together

Yields 2 servings

Basic Dressing

This is a common dressing from a basic Ann Wigmore kitchen.

1 celery stalk, chopped
¼ cup chives or scallions, chopped
½ teaspoon lemon juice
1 tablespoon sauerkraut
1 cup seed yogurt

In a glass mixing bowl, combine all ingredients and mix well. See the cultured foods section on page 95 for the veggie kraut and seed yogurt instructions.

Yields 2 servings

Carrot Ginger Dressing

¼ cup carrot juice
1 tablespoon celery powder or dulse (optional)
1 teaspoon lemon juice
1 teaspoon ginger, grated
1 teaspoon stevia leaves, chopped (optional)

Blend all ingredients into a delicious dressing.

Yields 2 servings

Use this dressing with moderation because of the high sugar content in carrot juice.

This is a tasty dressing which you will be able to tolerate if you are not severely invaded by Candida.

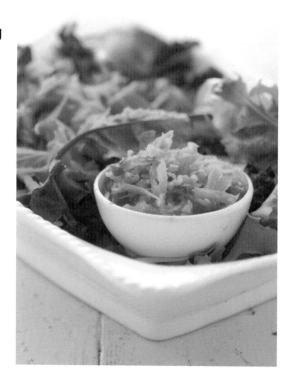

Milk

Seed Milk

1 cup soaked and sprouted
      sunflower or pumpkin seeds
2 cups rejuvelac or pure water
green stevia powder to taste (optional)

Blend ingredients and strain through a nut milk bag. This mixture will last up to 1 day.

Almond Milk

1 cup soaked almonds (peeling the almonds is optional for nut milk)
2 cups rejuvelac or pure water
green stevia powder to taste (optional)

Blend ingredients and strain through a nut milk bag. This mixture will last up to 1 day.

*You can soak and sprout your seeds then dehydrate them and store refrigerated in a sealed glass jar. This method will save you time when you need milk in a hurry, but of course it is best to use freshly soaked and sprouted seeds when they hold their optimal vitality.

Milk

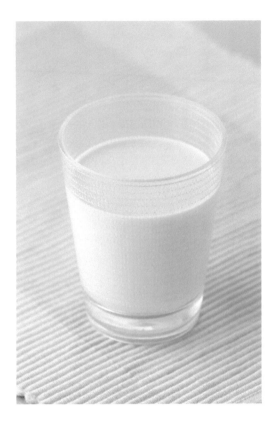

You can modify the milk consistency by adjusting the amount of liquid you use.

If you prefer a thicker more creamy milk, add less liquid (1 – 1 ½ cups). For a thinner consistency to your milk, add more liquid (2 ½ cups).

*Turn your milk into a creamy fruit drink by blending the strained milk with your favorite berries.

Cultured Foods

In general, cultured or fermented foods are a good source of vitamins B, C, and E. Cultured foods are rich in enzymes, easy to digest, and are one of the best sources of friendly bacteria (lactobacilli) which is very important to our digestive and elimination system. Replenishing our lactobacilli supply will help improve digestion and prevent constipation, thus supporting our colon health and promoting longevity. Fermented cabbage (sauerkraut and rejuvelac) is a source of natural vitamin C and highly recommended to reduce polyps, parasitic colon worms, and stomach ulcers. Sauerkraut will also naturally help the body decrease or increase the acidity in the stomach by balancing the levels of hydrochloric acid. Sauerkraut also produces lactic acid which is valuable in balancing the pH of the colon.

It is very important to have clean supplies when preparing any type of cultured foods so you do not jeopardize the success of your efforts. Remember the intent of culturing is to grow bacteria. The "good" bacteria will over power any "bad" bacteria that may try to reproduce, however if the preparation equipment (jars, bowls, mesh, juicer or blender) are not properly cleaned, unfriendly bacteria can reproduce and spoil your entire batch.

"Any cleansing program should begin with the colon...The main purpose of consuming fiber is elimination. Without fiber, complete elimination is nearly impossible, if possible at all." ***Bernard Jensen, D.C., Ph.D.***

Cultured Foods

Quinoa Rejuvelac

To make Rejuvelac you will need a large glass jar (one gallon size will do), mesh and a rubber band to hold it in place over the jar or a sprout bag.

Start by cleaning / rinsing sprouted Quinoa 3 times.

1 cup quinoa, sprouted
Water

Place the Quinoa in a clean glass jar; add water to the jar covering the Quinoa with 2 times the amount of water. Cover the jar with mesh or a sprout bag and allow the mixture to stand at room temperature for approximately 48 hours. Again the fermentation process will vary depending on temperature.

Strain off the liquid Rejuvelac into a fresh glass container and serve. The refrigerated Rejuvelac will keep for up to 5 days.

For a second batch: Leaving the Quinoa Seeds In the original jar covered with the liquid rejuvelac, add more water. Again covering the quinoa with 2 times the amount of water and covering with a mesh bag or sprout bag. Allow the second batch to sit for approximately 24 hours depending on the temperature.

Cabbage Rejuvelac

3 cups coarsely chopped, loosely packed fresh cabbage
1 ¾ cups water

Blend the cabbage and water and transfer to a jar; cover with mesh or a sprout bag and allow to stand at room temperature for 3 days.

Strain off the liquid Rejuvelac into a fresh glass container and serve. Refrigerated Rejuvelac will keep for up to 5 days.

It took me many years before I fully realized what I could do to help myself. Not only was I able to overcome my health problems, but I realized that when one turns to nature for help, there is seemingly no problem that cannot be solved. Now at age 82, I have more abundant energy than I have ever had.
– Ann Wigmore – Rebuild Your Health

Veggie Kraut

To make Veggie Kraut you will need an Omega or Champion Juicer with a blank plate, a large glass container (tall and narrow like a crock is the best) and a cloth mesh large enough to cover the container. Again, make sure your supplies are very clean so you do not jeopardize the success of your project.

1 head of cabbage (red or green)

Remove and save 3 – 5 cabbage leaves to use later as a cover. Optionally you can replace up to 20% of the cabbage with other vegetables such as cauliflower, carrots, broccoli or seaweed. Process the cabbage and other vegetables through the juicer using the blank plate. Place the mixture into the glass container pressing down to remove air pockets and to allow the juice to rise to the top. Make sure your container allows room for expansion. Cover the mixture with the stored cabbage leaves pressing down to seal the mixture. Cover with a mesh cloth and allow the mixture to stand at room temperature for 3 days.

If you are using other vegetables, layer the mixture for the best fermentation results. With broccoli and cauliflower you can cut the florets and set aside not passing through the juicer. When transferring to the fermenting container layer the cabbage, vegetables, and florets. Continue layering making sure the cabbage is the first and last layer as it is the cabbage that causes the fermentation or culturing process.

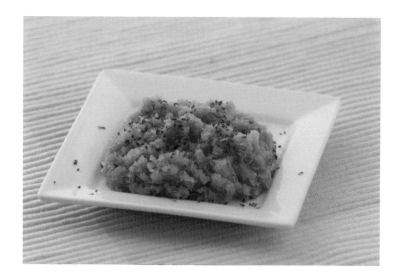

Cultured Foods

Seed Cheese

1 cup sunflower or pumpkin seeds, soaked and sprouted
> or

1 cup almonds, soaked and peeled
1 cup rejuvelac

Soak and sprout the seeds. If you are using nuts soak the nuts rinsing twice a day, if you are unable to rinse twice, soak the nuts in the refrigerator to prevent premature fermentation. See the Sprouting section on page 107 for directions on soaking and peeling almonds.

Yields 2 ½ cups

Cheese Using a Bag

Mix and blend the liquid with the seeds or nuts until it reaches a smooth paste texture. Pour the paste mixture into a sprout bag and hang over a bowl or sink for 3 – 8 hours (depending on the room temperature).

Remove the cheese from the bag and place in a glass container. Store tightly covered in the refrigerator.

Cheese Using a Jar

Mix and blend the liquid with the seeds or nuts until it reaches a smooth paste texture. Pour the paste mixture into a jar and cover with a mesh, cheesecloth or sprout bag and allow to stand for 3 – 8 hours (depending on the room temperature).

After the time has elapsed, use a spoon to remove the seed cheese from the jar without mixing it with the whey from the bottom of the jar. Put in a glass container and store tightly covered in the refrigerator. The whey or milk can be used in a dressing or in energy soup.

*note: Cheese will last in the refrigerator for 3 to 5 days. The cheese may turn a little bit darker but otherwise should not change color, taste or odor. If it does it should be discarded.

Address your health before it addresses you! It is not too late to turn an unhealthy lifestyle into a healthy alternative way of life. Give your body the nourishment it needs to become the self healing organism that God intended it to be.

Cultured Foods

Yogurt

The Yogurt recipe is very similar to making cheese, however we use slightly more liquid and mix in the whey or milk rather than being careful to skim the mixture from the top.

1 cup sunflower or pumpkin seeds, soaked and sprouted
    or
1 cup almonds, soaked and peeled
1 ¼ cup Rejuvelac (for a less dense yogurt add more liquid)

Soak and sprout the seeds. If you are using nuts, soak the nuts rinsing twice a day. If you are unable to rinse twice, soak the nuts in the refrigerator to prevent premature fermentation. *note: After soaking, the almonds must be peeled for this recipe.

Mix and blend the liquid with the seeds or nuts until it reaches a smooth paste texture. Pour the paste mixture into a glass jar or glass bowl and cover with a mesh, cheesecloth or sprout bag and let sit for 3 – 8 hours (depending on the room temperature.

As the ingredients separate the whey will settle to the bottom of your container. After the proper fermentation time has elapsed, using a spoon, mix the liquid whey with the more solid yogurt. Refrigerate in a tightly sealed glass container for up to 5 days.

Yields 3 cups

See the Sprouting section on page 107 for directions on soaking and peeling almonds.

Equipment List

Blender: One of the most important pieces of equipment in a raw kitchen along with a good set of sharp knives and a food processor is a good heavy duty blender. This should be one of the first purchases you make if you do not already have one. A good blender can save you time and frustration. A smaller lightweight blender will work but it will not have the capacity to prepare the quantities you need in a single batch. Some lighter weight blenders will not get the consistency you need. As an example, when preparing energy soup in a smaller blender you may have to blend the greens much longer to get the proper consistency. Over blended greens become bitter, giving your soup a bitter and unpleasant taste; not to mention what over blending of these delicate greens can do to the enzyme content. If using a light weight blended try to avoid over processing by taking advantage of the pulse mode. I personally like the Vita-Mix however there are other good quality blenders out there.

Cutting Boards: Invest in one or two good cutting boards if you do not already have one. I use a large size for cutting up the medium to large fruits and vegetables and a smaller one for the smaller produce. In Puerto Rico we use glass or plastic, but many people from cooler climates prefer the wooden boards.

Citrus Juicer: I like to have a citrus juicer on hand because many of the recipes I use call for lemon juice. A standard juicer will work but I find the manual hand held citrus juicer much easier if I simply need a small amount of lemon juice for a recipe.

103

Equipment List

Coffee Grinder: This can be used for grinding seeds or nuts when only small amounts are needed. A dry blender will work in most cases but a coffee grinder is easier for small amounts.

Dehydrator: With a dehydrator the most important feature is a temperature control. It is very important with Living Foods to keep them alive to preserve the Enzymes. It has been scientifically documented that enzymes begin to be destroyed at 118F. As a precautionary measure we never have the temperature over 115F.

Glass Jars: The glass jars could be replaced with crocks, but I find the one gallon glass jars the best for making Rejuvelac. Glass jars or crocks also seem to be the best choice for making sauerkraut.

Glass Mixing Bowls: I recommend a variety of glass mixing bowls for meal preparation. I prefer glass or ceramic bowls for food preparation. I do not recommend using plastic for food preparation or for food storage or serving. If you do use ceramic, make sure it has not been chemically treated.

Food Processor: A food processor is very useful when preparing larger quantities of fruits, vegetables, or nuts. Some people use a food processor and a blender interchangeably and that will work, however there are some dishes that are just better in a blender and some that turn out better with a food processor. I have listed in each recipe if the ingredients should be processed or blended so you can get the best results.

Juicer: A good juicer is very important in a raw kitchen. I recommend purchasing an Omega or Champion juicer for these recipes. With either of these juicers you can make fruit or vegetable juice as well as use them with the blank plate for making sauerkraut, pâté, ice cream or other raw food treats. The Champion is a little easier to setup and clean however, the Omega gives you the option of juicing leafy greens which the Champion is not capable of. It really depends what you plan to use the juicer for, but either will work for any recipe in this book that calls for a juicer.

Knives: If you do not have good quality knives I would recommend purchasing some. If you can afford them, ceramic knives are the best for cutting fruits and vegetables but there are many other good knives available. At the minimum you should have a very good paring knife and a sharp, sturdy vegetable knife. It will save time and also save you a level of frustration if you have good knives to work with.

Nut Milk and Sprout Bags: Nut Milk and Sprout Bags are separate items. Each is important and in most cases should not be used interchangeably. The Nut Milk bag has a much smaller screen and is needed when you filter or press the nuts and seeds from the milk. A Sprout Bag can be replaced with a mesh screen but in some cases like when you are preparing cheese, a Sprout Bag is just easier to work with.

Spiral Slicer or Mandolin: I use the spiral slicer or mandolin to make zucchini spaghetti and to make decorative vegetables or fruits for decorative platters. Shredded zucchini spaghetti made in the food processor will work just fine, however a spiral slicer gives the zucchini a much more authentic spaghetti look and feel.

Sprouting Chart

Soaking and Sprouting is necessary for all Nuts and Seeds. Along with providing easier to digest nourishment that can be assimilated into the body with much less effort, the soaking and sprouting process has many additional benefits.

Sprouting Benefits:
- Release Enzyme Inhibitors
- Increase Vitamin & Mineral Content
- Produce More Alkaline Forming Food
- Turn Protein into Amino Acids
- Turn Carbohydrates into Simple Sugars
- Turn Fats into Fatty Acids
- Provide a High Quality Protein Food
- Produce a Less Mucus Forming Food

To soak seeds, nuts, or grains place in a glass jar or bowl covering with twice the amount of water then cover the container with a mesh or sprout bag. Allow to soak for the directed time (see the sprout chart on the following page).

When soaking almonds; change the water and rinse at least twice a day. If you are not able to rinse them twice a day, soak in the refrigerator to prevent premature fermentation. (Almonds do not sprout or produce a tail.)

Sprouting time will vary depending on temperature and altitude.

To sprout seeds, place them in a sprout bag or in a glass jar positioned at an angle over a drain board for the directed amount of time. The seeds should be rinsed during the sprouting process 2 or 3 times a day. If you can not rinse as often as recommended; sprout in a jar to prevent loss of moisture. Again, if you can not rinse the seeds or grains at all, you will have to sprout in the refrigerator. Refrigerated sprouting is not as fast as room temperature, but it will work.

Supplies Needed:

- Pure Water for Soaking and Rinsing
- A Glass or Ceramic Jar or Bowl
- A Mesh Cloth or Sprout Bag

The Ann Wigmore Institute is very selective with the types of nuts, seeds, and grains that we use based on safety and nutritional value. For example, we do not endorse the use of pine nuts because we have found them to be too oily and can become rancid in a very short time. Included on our "never use list" are walnuts, cashews and peanuts because they have a tendency to carry such a high mold content that we feel they are not safe for human consumption.

Peeling Almonds:

Peeling almonds is a simple task that can be made more simplistic by simple placing the soaked almonds in warm water just prior to peeling. The warmed almonds can be squeezed out of the peel by rubbing two almonds together or by rubbing them with a dish towel.

Sprouting Chart

This is not a complete sprouting chart because I choose to include only seeds, nuts and grains that are recommended for Candida friendly recipes.

Type	Soak Hrs	Sprout Time	Tail Length / Size of Seed
Almonds	12 - 48	Does not sprout	
Amaranth	6 – 8	1 – 2 Days	1 – 3 x's
Buckwheat grouts	½ - 1	2 Days	1 -3 x's
Flax seed	6 – 8	Do not sprout	See note above
Lentils	6 - 8	2 – 3 Days	¼" – ¾" or 4 - 5- x's
Pumpkin	6 – 8	2 – 4 Hours	0"- 1/8"
Quinoa	6 - 8	14 – 16 Hours	1 – 3 x's
Sunflower	6 – 8	2 – 4 Hours	0" – 1/8"

Remember that sprouting time will vary depending on the temperature and humidity. The warm humid tropical weather in Puerto Rico allows a shorter sprouting time than in a cooler and less humid environment.

Note: At the Ann Wigmore Institute we do not sprout Flax seed as they are too oily and very sensitive to temperatures. We find the sprouting process can cause premature fermentation.

Testimonials

Psoriasis: After going to dermatologists for about a year I realized that their help was not much help at all. Every appointment was the same thing: "There is no cure for psoriasis; you're going to have to deal with this for the rest of your life. Here are some creams that might help the itching."

I was feeling so depressed that I was almost ready to start taking anti-depressants. But I'm the type of person who will not give up when something is in the way of my health. Finding their help unsatisfactory I began to look for alternative ways to solve my problem. I started to look into different diets, while doing so, I found Lalita Salas. Unlike the dermatologists, the first thing she said was "We're going to get rid of this". Lalita gave me a diet to follow and after following her recommended diet for about a week I felt different, I was more optimistic and I didn't feel so depressed all the time. About twenty days into the diet, I was already seeing results on my skin. What the "specialists" told me would stay with me forever was healing in a matter of weeks.

Thank you Lalita for coming my way,
Florencia Fridman
Ridgewood, NJ
USA

Testimonials

Systemic Candida Overgrowth: I'm just back from my second stay at the Ann Wigmore Institute where I continued my study of the Living Foods Lifestyle with Lalita Salas. I've fallen in love with this lifestyle, it relieved me of a systemic Candida overgrowth that was manifesting a number of debilitating symptoms ranging from skin rashes, blinding headaches, insomnia, indigestion, depression, and lethal crankiness. I had tried everything else, including western medicine, the standard Candida diet, and a fortune in natural supplements. With these methods I had experienced some improvement; but nothing completely relieved the condition or my symptoms until my stay at the Institute. For any physical dysfunction the Ann Wigmore Institute is now the first place I'd head.

The benefits of the Living Foods Lifestyle go way beyond the alleviation of Candida overgrowth. There are other benefits one might expect to experience such as weight loss, rejuvenation, an increase in energy; and as I'm beginning to discover, there are the hidden benefits like greater mental clarity, a calmer and more patient outlook on life, a lightness of spirit, joy in simplicity, and also inspiration, particularly, for one like myself who loves food, in the alchemical potential of live fruits and vegetables. Truly, I do not exaggerate.

Thank you Lalita and Thank You to the Ann Wigmore Institute!
Love Susan Ray
USA

Testimonials

Rheumatoid Arthritis: Over the last 32 years, I have been ill, except for a 6 year remission period. It all started in October of 1972, when a vaginal infection was treated with antibiotics, a Candida outbreak followed. From 1993 to 2006, I was on cortisone. In addition, I was prescribed sulfonamide between May 2004 and December 2006 for the treatment of intestinal staphylococcus and in December of 2006, after 6 months of diarrhea, test results showed the presence of Candida. Before arriving at the Ann Wigmore Institute in Puerto Rico on January 14, 2007, I was taking 2 anti-inflammatory pills and 3 doses of paracetamol (antipyretic and analgesic) with codeine per day. Regardless of all these treatments, my body was in terrible pain. Nights were literally a nightmare; any movement would result in excruciating pain.

For the trip to Puerto Rico from Europe, I used a morphine patch to help make my travels more bearable. On January 20, 2007, six days after arriving at Ann Wigmore, I stopped all medication. On February 27, 2007, I estimate that the pain was reduced by about 50%. The only way I can think to describe it is that I it feels like I'm coming out of hell. I strongly intend to stay on living foods at 100%.

Thank you Lalita, Leola, and all the team, you are wonderful and loving and you saved my life.
Isabelle – 59 years young
France

Closing Thoughts

The process to adopt a new lifestyle can seem very complicated to people. We grow up feeling and understanding the "perfect" order in the food we eat. We are blind to the chaos that is going on inside our bodies that we human beings created with our preservatives, colorants, and genetically modified foods.

This food that is perfect for our conditioned minds but so out of balance for our natural bodies that we are not able to feel the chaos that develops subtly until one day we "catch" some type of condition or pain that screams at us for attention.

It is incredible how we can understand in our minds but not really accept deep inside our consciousness or natural state of being. We are not connected or in tune with who and what our bodies want and need therefore seem to respond, eat, and live according to years of accumulated "knowledge" and ideas with our preconceived thought process on how things "should" be. We are so far removed from the natural beings we really are that we no longer recognize the law of nature nor can we function in harmony with it." **–Lalita Salas**

"The body truly is a self-healer. You have a doctor within that is capable of healing the body through self-responsibility. You simply need to provide the body with the proper tools in the form of living easy-to-digest nourishment, and provide an environment for rebuilding health. This is extremely important and it is possible."
–Dr. Ann Wigmore; Rebuild Your Health

Acknowledgments

Many people throughout my life have inspired me to write this book, when I think about it, it seems as though in some subtle way most of my life's experiences have guided me to share this knowledge with as many people as possible.

First and foremost I am grateful to Michele Jarvey who has been a co-creator of this book. I kept saying that I would like to write a book to help people with Candida but that was as far as it went. She gently pushed me to work on this book, giving me a starting point and patiently organizing the material into a book format. Michele trusted in me and when I became discouraged, she helped me get back on track, encouraging me with her patience, faith and love.

My dear friend Leola Brooks, has been my partner, teacher, friend and sister in the Living Foods Lifestyle for 16 years. With her wisdom and love, Leola has inspired me and given me the strength and courage to write this book. Thank you Leola for everything you are and everything you have done to help me see this book to completion.

I am indebted to my husband Héctor for his patience with everything I do. Thank you Héctor for always being there for me with your unconditional love and support throughout the years but especially during this journey I have taken us on toward balance and optimal health.

Acknowledgments

I am thankful for my children with their seemingly endless questions as they were growing up. Their open and honest questioning about many things in life helped me to wake up to the realities involved with the natural balancing act that a healthy terrain provides.

The innocent faces and purity of love that my grandchildren freely display has been such an inspiration for me. Their innocence and trust has been an inspiration for me to learn, live, and teach everyone that wants to live a healthier lifestyle.

I extend my gratitude to my children-in-laws for the respect and appreciation they have shown to me.

I will be eternally grateful to all the students that come through the program at AWNHI; their love, curiosity, disappointments, and seemingly endless faith has been a daily inspiration to me.

I wish to acknowledge all the staff at AWNHI for all the support they gave me during myself experimentation; but especially the kitchen for giving extra care with all my energy soup trials and the agriculture department for providing such a variety of greens.

I wish a special thank you to the Ann Wigmore teachers that supported me with this project in different ways.

I also want to acknowledge my dear friend and teacher Tao Becker, my first Living Foods teacher, to Sandra, for encouraging me to write about my personal struggle, to Carolyn for supporting me during my first attempt at cleansing my Candida overgrowth and to my friend Anandi and her young daughter Francesca for inspiring me with their love and dedication to health.

Acknowledgments

And last but not least I would like to thank our chef Manuel Acevedo; this book would not be possible without his help. Manuel was so patient with the demands I put on him while we were perfecting the recipes. Often he had to repeat a recipe several times as I made minor alterations trying to achieve the perfect taste or texture. Manuel never complained nor did he ever become impatient with the process. He added his creative touch and chef's intuition to the recipes and for this I thank him very much.

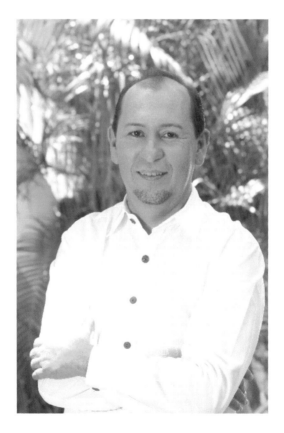

"Living foods brought light into my life."
--Manuel Acevedo

Author's Note

According to the psychiatrist Laurence J. Bendit; Healing is basically the result of putting right our wrong relation to our body, to other people and...to our own complicated minds, with their emotions and instincts at war with one another and not properly understood or accepted by what we call "I" or "me". The process is one of reorganization, reintegration of things which have come apart.

I love this definition because it reminds me of Candida overgrowth. When we suffer from Candida we are not in tune with our inner selves and can not organize our Lifestyle to be in harmony with our body, our emotions, or our food.

If you are ready to enter the path of healing, let's talk about the total solution to restoring your body's delicate micro-ecological balance with food, exercise, colon cleansing and a positive mental attitude. As you will discover while reading this book, the solution is not so difficult. But remember, we must start by developing patience and a deep love for ourselves. During this adventure we are going to reverse the aging process of being composted and recycled and begin enjoying total wellbeing while unlocking the abundant energy that our body holds inside.

We must nourish our bodies with essential vitamins, minerals and other elements obtained from the appropriate foods prepared and eaten in the proper manner, or our body will never be strong enough to take over on its own.

To enjoy optimal health and an abundance of energy, I recommend Living Foods, but if you are still eating cooked food, I recommend a gentle and healthy transition. Start by removing Candida promoting foods and gradually incorporating more Living Foods into your Lifestyle. Start out slowly by adding 25% of Living Foods until it becomes part of your normal daily routine, then increase it to 50%, then 75% striving to reach the magic number of 100%. Please be gentle and loving yet firm with yourself and your plans to achieve the perfect balance. Only you have the power to incorporate these healthy changes and start living the healthy life that you deserve.

During this transition it is important to do some type of exercise like yoga, walking or aerobics, and do not forget the importance of deep breathing for at least 5 minutes every day, gradually increasing the time. (Deep breathing can help relax you at a cellular level.)

Take pleasure with nature as much as you can, find time to be outside in the fresh air at least one hour each day. Enjoy a sunset, a sunrise, or a full moon every day. Try to walk barefoot on green grass or on a sandy beach at least three times a week. Read books that inspire you to be in contact with your inner self and that will help you understand the cleansing process which your body is going through. Seek out other health conscious people, explain to your friends and relatives about your new way of living and ask for their support without imposing your new Lifestyle on them.

Most importantly remember to be loving and gentle with yourself not only during this process but always as part of your new and healthful lifestyle.

Author's Note

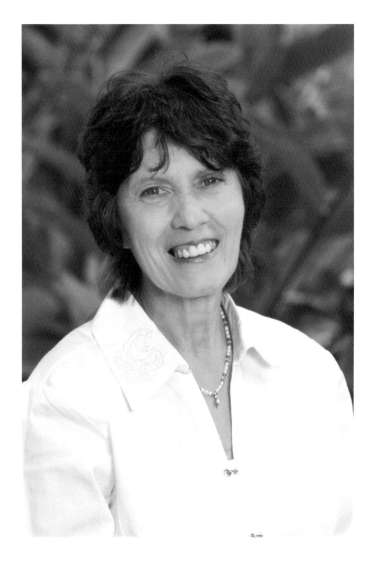

Wishing you health, love and balance,

Lalita Salas

About Ann Wigmore

Ann Wigmore was born in Lithuania in 1909 where her grandmother raised her until the age of 16 when she joined her parents in the United States. In 1963 she opened the Hippocrates Institute in Boston, Massachusetts which was the first holistic health institute of its type in the United States. That institute was appropriately named after the Father of Medicine whose recommended cure for disease was water, fresh air and sunshine. Ann Wigmore believed, taught, and lived Hippocrates teachings; "Let food be your medicine". The Hippocrates Institute later became the Ann Wigmore Foundation and has since relocated to San Fidel, New Mexico.

In 1990 she founded the Ann Wigmore Natural Health Institute in Aguada, Puerto Rico where she continued her studies and refinement of the Living Foods Lifestyle, which is still taught there today in its purest form. The Institute is a non-profit school dedicated to continue the teachings of Dr. Ann Wigmore's Living Foods Lifestyle. Through this simple natural lifestyle, people from all walks of life have taken control of their lives and their health.

Ann Wigmore; Teacher, Healer, Living Foods Lifestyle® Founder and Author of numerous books and articles on Living Foods, dedicated her life to educating the world about the transforming qualities of this wonderful lifestyle.

About Ann Wigmore

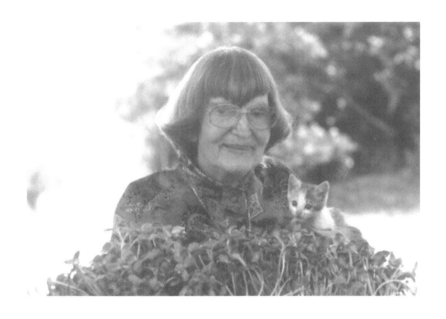

"As you enter into a healthy lifestyle, using easy-to-digest nourishment, you begin to feel that you can overcome even these so called incurable conditions which have previously been very stressful for you to deal with."
–Dr. Ann Wigmore

References

"The Body Ecology Diet"-Donna Gates with Linda Schatz

"Candida Albicans"-Ray C. Wenderlich, Jr., MD & Dwight K. Kalita PhD

"Healing with Whole Foods" Third Edition-Paul Pitchford -

"Hooked on Raw"-Rhio

"Optimal Wellness"-Ralph Golan, MD

"Rainbow Green Live-Food Cuisine"-Gabriel Cousens, MD

"Think Before You Eat"-Diane Olive,

Attend classes with Lalita Salas at

The Ann Wigmore Natural Health Institute
Aguada, Puerto Rico

Phone: 787.868.6307

info@annwigmore.org

www.annwigmore.org

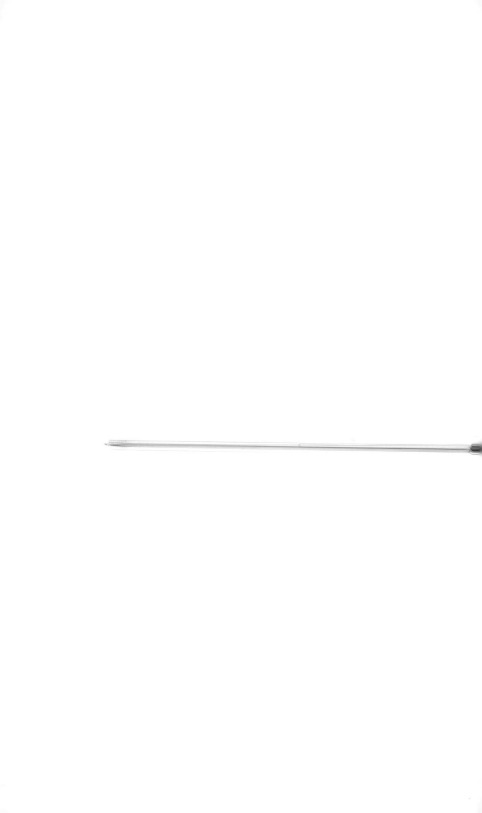

LaVergne, TN USA
24 September 2009
158937LV00001BA